NOW WHAT?

A Guide for Men Starting Over in Life After
Infidelity, Breakup and Divorce

BY D.S.O.

www.dadstartingover.com

Thank you, Button.

Contents

CONTENTS

Prologue
"I have to be the dumbest fucking idiot on the planet."

Steve's email was very typical for readers of my site at dadstartingover.com. All of the situations are roughly the same, yet they all think they're unique in their own special blend of *"stupid"*. Steve, like many other readers, was convinced that the entire world was in on a cosmic joke at his expense. He feels like Jim Carrey's character from *"The Truman Show"*. Unbeknownst to him, everyone around him was a cast member of a secret TV show... and the whole world was watching and laughing. He just pulled back the curtain and everything is finally starting to make sense. He doesn't like what he sees. It was all just a big charade. Nothing was ever real.

Over the last few months, he has run the events that led him to this point again and again in his mind. He's trying to figure out where the marriage machine broke down. Dammit, he did everything by the fucking book and yet his marriage sure didn't go as planned. Not at all. He was promised a better life than this. He was promised the wife, the kids, the grandkids and the picket fence. He was promised comfort and stability. He did his part, god damnit, why didn't she?!

Now he's in an empty apartment, driving a shitty old Ford pickup truck that breaks down half the time, and he's only allowed to see his kids on Wednesdays after school and every other weekend. This really really sucks and it doesn't look like it's going to get any better in the foreseeable future.

The TV show audience is now pointing and laughing at him. *"Haha!! He bought into the whole 'Til death do us part' thing?! Haha!! What a dumbass!"* Steve is now a dangerous combination of angry, hurt, scared, and confused.

1

"I'm a Good Guy! I Swear!"

Most readers in Steve's shoes will immediately start to list all of the positive stuff they did in their marriage. Steve was no different.

"I did laundry, I cooked, I cleaned, I did it all. I paid all the bills while she went into huge amounts of debt for her degree. I didn't complain fucking once. I supported her in everything. She doesn't give a shit about anything I did for her."

Steve was building up a *"Good Provider"* resume for me so that I wouldn't think he was some abusive asshole loser like *"most other guys"* are. In his mind, he checked ALL of the *"good husband"* boxes. To think that his wife would even consider stepping outside of their marriage never occurred to him, but, that's exactly what she did. Multiple times.

The first time it happened, he saw text messages between her and a guy from her work. Steve had his suspicions. He saw her strange behavior going on for weeks. One evening, he finally got a hold of her phone and read every one of their messages to each other. He saw how the conversation and their relationship got progressively more sexual as time went on. He saw pictures that they sent back and forth. At first, their messages were innocent and friendly. Then they weren't. He couldn't believe what he was looking at. THIS was his loving wife?

He went to the internet for help. A quick Google search gave him pages and pages of results. He read up on the growing phenomenon of *"emotional affairs"* that were happening more and more thanks to social media and websites like Facebook. Steve read what to do if you catch your wife in this scenario, and he followed the advice to the letter. He approached his wife and her new

2

boyfriend and stopped the emotional affair dead in its tracks.

The second affair occurred with an old boyfriend from her pre-marriage past. He was the quintessential *"one that got away"*. For years she would send innocent Facebook messages to him on every birthday and every Christmas, just so he wouldn't forget she was still around. Steve knew about this ex-boyfriend, but he wasn't worried. This guy had his own wife and three kids, and he lived really far away, so he was nothing to really worry about. Steve was convinced that his wife's cheating days were well behind her. They both put in a lot of work over the years and really grew together as a couple. Through good times and bad, they were a team.

After one typical *"Merry Christmas!"* message from the wife to the ex-boyfriend, he responded unusually. "*I really miss you. I think about you a lot.*" That set off a chain reaction in Steve's wife. Those old lustful feelings came right back. Their conversation went from sappy to sexual in no time. They remembered all the dirty escapades they had together all those many years ago. Two hours into their heated conversation, they made plans to meet. The ex-boyfriend left his wife and kids for a *"business trip"* and drove eight hours to see Steve's wife. Steve's wife simply had to skip her university classes for a day. She told a female classmate what she was up to and they both agreed on a cover story to use in case anyone asked where she was. She promised to pay her friend back with dinner and drinks.

The two old lovers finally met. They spent hours reconnecting and having sex. Old feelings came right back. It was like the years apart just melted away. They both envisioned a long and wild love affair that would give them much-needed relief from their respective boring marriages and god-awful home life. They were both equally sick of screaming kids and the dull spouses they lost attraction to years ago.

Unbeknownst to his wife, Steve knew ALL the details of this latest secret affair. He had been tracking her exact whereabouts and all of her online activity for several weeks now. Thanks to all the tricks he learned on the internet, he had become quite the private investigator and knew exactly how to get ahold of her conversations without her knowing. The dummy forgot she was logged into Facebook on an old laptop they had lying around. Steve would sometimes watch their conversations happening in real time.

Before he started spying on his wife again, he conferred with his friends. Was he just being paranoid? They all agreed that yes, he was acting crazy. He should respect his wife's privacy, they told him. That emotional affair of hers was YEARS ago, and she's been a great wife to him. He kept telling them that something just didn't feel right. She was acting like her old cheater self again.

Unfortunately, his gut was right and his friends were wrong.

Again, thanks to the internet, he knew exactly what to do next. He was going to do all he could to ruin his wife and her lover. He was a man on a mission.

- He informed the lover's spouse of the affair.
- He told the lover's employer why he missed work.
- He told officials at his wife's school that she was missing classes and why.
- He met with an attorney and drew up a plan for splitting assets and debts.
- He filed for divorce right away.

Steve would learn what most men in his situation learn:

Nobody gives a shit.

His wife's lover wasn't fired. He kept his job. He's since been promoted. He's even still married to the same woman. Absolutely nothing has changed for the cheating bastard. His wife actually got angry at Steve when he called her with evidence of her husband's affair. She bluntly told him to stay out of her life and never contact her again. Steve would later learn that his wife's lover was quite the player. This was not his first affair rodeo, and the wife sticks by him through it all.

The university administrative office never even replied to his repeated emails and calls. His wife would later brag to him that she was friends with the office staff, and they all just laughed at his crazy emails and calls. They called him *"that psycho husband"*. They couldn't care less about a student's personal love life or if she skipped classes. What does that have to do with them? As long as she keeps paying the bills for the classes, his wife can skip however many classes and screw around with whoever she wants. After a while, the university eventually sent him an email and let him know that his personal matters have nothing to do with the school and to please stop harassing them or they will be forced to contact the police.

When it came time to divorce, it went a lot rougher than what Steve anticipated. His wife's family, the ones he considered the surrogate parents that he loved with all his heart, cut off all contact with him. He considered this one of the largest acts of betrayal he had ever seen. *"Mom and dad"* abandoned him in favor of their *"whore daughter"*. He was a great husband to their daughter and a great son-in-law to them. They didn't care one bit. They stuck the knife in even further when they helped his wife pay for a really good attoney. This was a really good attorney with a reputation for getting divorced moms a lot of money. The attorney would live up to his reputation.

Steve was painted as the villain in court documents. The words *"abusive"* and *"neglect"* came up more than once. He was baffled. None of this was true. He was a good man. A good husband. A good father. Why would they do this to him?

Steve's own lawyer was nowhere near as well-seasoned as his wife's attorney. Yes, the wife's affair was brought up, but thanks to **"no-fault"** laws, it had zero bearing on much of anything. In the end, it was just a matter of who should have the kids and when, who gets what asset, and who gets stuck with what bill.

After all was said and done, Steve was left in a small apartment on the opposite side of town with a growing stack of bills, half his 401k, zero savings, and a new drinking habit. Understandably, he feels that the world has just chewed him up and spit him out. The second he tried to make his case and prove his worth as a man, the world laughed at his naivety.

That's when Steve ended up on my website.

I patiently scroll and read page after page of his first email to me. This is nothing new. I'm no longer shocked. I've officially heard it all. This is actually not THAT bad of a case compared to some I have read._At least one of his ex-wife's mentally ill lovers didn't stab him nine times in the back and leave him to die like the other guy I recently talked to.

After a few emails back and forth, with Steve saying over and over that this isn't how it was supposed to turn out…I grow a little impatient and say what I say to all guys in his position:

"Okay. You were wrong. Now what?"

It's Time to Rebuild

When you join the military, they send you to boot camp. Based on what branch of the military you are in; they are all varying degrees of an extremely strenuous experience that few recruits are mentally and physically prepared for. All of these boot camps have the same end result in mind: They want to break you down and completely rebuild you from the ground up. Why? Because it works.

They don't want a soldier with baggage. They don't want a soldier with a mental catalog of self-limiting thoughts and behaviors. They don't want a soldier who *"triggers"* and cries when something very stressful and dangerous is going on around them. They want a machine. They want a machine that reacts in the way that will keep themselves and their fellow soldiers alive and still able to carry out the mission. That's it.

This is the mindset of truly starting over. This is what *"Now What?"* is all about.

It's time to break you down and REBUILD you from the ground up. If we're going to do this, we're going to do it right. No pussy-footing around. No dancing around your emotions. No telling you just what you want to hear to make you feel better. It's time to get to work.

Rebuilding is about setting aside all of the stupid BULLSHIT that happened to you before. It's about realizing you can be whoever and whatever the hell you want to be. I make it sound simple because it is. Technically, it's as easy as making the first step and saying *"I'm going to do this"* … then the rest falls into place. So many men can't even bring themselves to make that first step. It's absolutely terrifying.

If you're a man living in a free country and you have a functioning body and an average IQ, there's no reason you can't take the steps you need to turn the page on this god-awful chapter in your life. That's exactly what it is, after all: **One chapter in a much larger story.** This is something that HAPPENED to you, not something that has to DEFINE you. It's a part of your life story. Make it a springboard that launches you to better things or make it a giant mud pit of awfulness that continuously drags you down and eventually overwhelms you. Up to you, amigo.

Life fucked you over. *So... Now What?*

Who This Book is For

This book was written for heterosexual men that have endured a failed long-term relationship with a woman and are having a difficult time picking up the pieces and starting over in life. **This book will appeal especially to those men who have discovered that their wife committed infidelity.** For these men, life as they know it was completely turned upside down. I understand the confusion, the despair, and the anger that you are going through. I went through it all, too. You need a little help, a little boost, to help you understand it all and to get you up and over the wall. That's what this book is for.

Maybe you've never been married. Maybe you just had a long-term girlfriend that suddenly broke up with you and you're trying to understand what happened and how to successfully move forward. For you, consider this book a lesson in both why your breakup may have happened AND how you can avoid a ton of trouble with the women in your future (yes, there WILL be more women). Learn from all of us who have been there and done that. An ounce of prevention is worth a pound of cure, as they say.

In 2015, I started the website at **dadstartingover.com** as a way for me to write and talk about my experiences and my personal philosophies about relationships as I move forward in life. I continue to learn as I go. Creating the website and my regular articles were very much a form of therapy for me. Thankfully, I have received a healthy amount of emails and web traffic that continues to grow on a daily basis.

There was and continues to be a growing demand for the material on my site. At the time of this writing, dadstartingover. com is at or near the top of search results for popular terms like "dead bedrooms", "signs my wife cheated on me", and "wife wants open marriage". Thousands of men are online looking for answers they never thought they would need. Some men don't like what they read on my site. It cuts a little too close to the bone for them. It's not the warm and fuzzy solutions they were looking for. Yet, most men that contact me find the information valuable and eye-opening. The site gives them the extra oomph they need to come to terms with their situation and to begin the process of starting over.

Are you one of these men? You are not alone. Not by a longshot. Welcome to the club.

My Story

You hear it all the time: *"I remember it like it was yesterday."* It's true. With traumatic moments come crystal clear recollection. I remember all the sounds and smells of that day. This cruel photographic memory of traumatic events is there for a reason. I think of it as my brain's way of making sure I learned my lesson and never ever forget what happened. Don't worry, brain. I won't forget. Lesson learned.

I was on the beach in sunny Florida with my wife and three kids. Weather was perfect. The kids were having a blast making sand castles and running out into the ocean. Lots of laughs. This was a much-needed vacation for us. It's not like we had a really tough and strenuous life back home. It was mostly what I would later call a very "meh" existence. We lived for the kids. Both worked. That's it. We were not a very intimate couple at all. We were buddies living under the same roof. The vacation in Florida was something different to take our mind off the banality of our existence. School, soccer games, work, house cleaning, basketball games, more work, wrestling meets, more work, more cleaning. That was our life. Being a parent can be a real drag... and something simple like sitting on the beach and staring at the ocean can make you feel like you're alive again.

Our one-and-a-half-year-old baby boy was getting cranky. Nap time. I volunteered to take the boy up to the condo while mom stayed on the beach with the two older kids. My back was hurting and lying on the couch in the AC sounded nice at the time. I take the baby boy up, shower him off, put him to bed in fresh jammies, and lie down on the couch with the laptop to start surfing the web and possibly doze off.

I open up the laptop and the first thing I see is that the browser is open to Facebook. My wife is logged in. For some reason, and to this day I really don't know why, I decided to snoop. I went right to her messages, and there it was: A brief snippet of a conversation between her and her personal trainer (yes, it's every bit as cliched as it sounds). Their chat was sexual in nature, and obviously just a small part of a longer conversation. She had failed to delete these last few messages back and forth, but it was enough for me to see what was going on. She was having an affair. Busted.

I could go on and on about what happened next, but I will spare you the gory details. My marriage ended that day, and my wife was the one that threw in the dynamite and blew it all up. She filed for divorce right away. Like most of you reading this, I tried to reconcile and keep the family together. Every single thing I did was wrong and just made the situation even worse. I should've just walked away with my head held high. I didn't. I groveled. I became even less of a man in her eyes and in the eyes of everyone around me. I was pitiful. I was pitiful at home, I was pitiful at work and I was pitiful with friends. Nobody likes a pitiful man, as I was quick to learn. I lost a lot of respect from my social group during that time period and my relationships with them still aren't the same to this day.

My ex-wife was relieved that this deep dark secret of hers was finally out in the open and she was free to start this new and exciting chapter of her life. As for me, I was left wondering what in the hell had just happened and where exactly I was supposed to go next. After all, everything about me revolved around my wife and my kids. I had zero family in the state we lived in, hell, I had zero family in the whole entire country! All of my known blood relatives live in Europe. I did have a group of close friends, but they were all out of state. I left them behind when we moved to be closer to my wife's family. Everybody I knew in our little town was because of my wife. I was friends with her coworkers and their spouses, but nothing beyond that. I worked from home, so I didn't have coworker friends to fall back on like my wife did. I was not, and still am not, what you would call a "social butterfly". I'm a writer. A designer. A creative. I do greatly enjoy my measured doses of friend and party time. I can talk your head off, but I also enjoy my alone time. It keeps me sane. Ironically, that all went right out the fucking window with divorce.

I ended up with my kids 4 - 5 days a week, depending upon my ex's "work" schedule. Whether or not I had the temperament for the job didn't matter. I was now mom and dad. You see, for my ex, being a divorced mom with a new boyfriend took up a tremendous amount of her time and energy. It's hard to shoehorn kid time into your life when you're busy playing the mating game with a new partner. Her solution, more often than not, was to just leave the kids alone at her house, with friends, or with me. Being in love can make you do some stupid things, as we all know.

After the divorce, my ex became a completely new human being. That is not at all an exaggeration. There is very little of the woman I knew for 20 years still there. Physically, she is a new human (not in a good way), and behaviorally she's an exaggeration of all the negatives she and I both used to despise. She became exactly what she said she always hated. I would learn that this is common amongst broken adulterous women.

Was this person we see now always in there, lurking away in the shadows of her psychological baggage? Was the person I knew and loved just a facade all those years? Was she really molded and shaped that easily by her new man? What in the hell happened to my best friend?

In hindsight, I did a really shitty job of properly vetting my wife candidate. I let too much bullshit slip through the cracks over the years. I ignored the obvious red flags for the sake of being a faithful and loving husband. Yes, we did end up having three beautiful children together and I love them with all of my heart… but the result of my poor marital decisions is starting to show itself beyond just a cheating ex-wife and a divorce. My daughter's

13

emotional fragility and depression is a result of me not manning up and doing what was right early in the relationship game. My ex is a really messed up human being, so of course our daughter is a wreck, too.

Since going through this awful chapter of my life, I have learned a great deal about the relationship game, about starting over, and about myself. Going through it has been hell at times, but I wouldn't change anything. The pain has been a great learning experience and has helped shape me into the man I am today.

Much like my ex-wife, I am a completely different human being now… but in a good way. There is very little of the old me left.

Good riddance, I say. He was a dumb fuck, anyway.

PART ONE
RETHINKING RELATIONSHIPS

It's time to set aside all your preconceived notions about love and relationships. It's time to shed all your "nice guy" behaviors that probably got you into this mess in the first place. It's time to wipe the slate clean and look at this situation you're in with a new set of eyes.

This won't be pretty. This won't be nice. It will probably hurt quite a bit. All I can tell you is… it's the truth. The truth is, more often than not, ugly, but you have to embrace reality before you can move forward in life and make real progress. You need to know how you got here and how to stop yourself from ever being in this situation again.

Get ready, my friend. It's time to go down the rabbit hole of what relationships are really all about.

Chapter 1: Why Did This Happen?

Did you catch your wife or long-term girlfriend cheating on you? Maybe she just suddenly asked for some "space" or a "relationship timeout" so that she think clearly about your future together? Maybe she needs to go away and "find" herself. Did she say, *"I just don't have feelings for you anymore"* or *"I love you but I'm not IN LOVE with you"*? Did she just ask you for an open relationship? Sorry, my man. It's over.

All of these are the typical signs of cheating partner (we'll say "wife" to keep it simple). She has probably detached from you and latched onto another human being. Once that happens, there is no going back to your old life. The woman you knew and loved is dead.

I know, you can't believe it. You refuse to believe it. You don't want life as you knew it to be over. Not like this. It's all just happening way too fast for you to comprehend. I know you probably hold on to a glimmer of hope that your relationship with your ex will rekindle and it will be as strong as ever. You probably have fantasies of your ex "waking up" from this crazy irrational stupor she is in and suddenly remembering what a great couple you are and recognizing the value in the life you have built together over all these years. *"I don't know what I was thinking. I love you!! Let's start over again!"*

There are lots of friends, therapists and others that will sell you on the dream of reconciliation. I'm not one of them. I've literally never seen reconciliation succeed long-term after a wife's affair. It's most likely just not going to happen for you. I'm sorry. I know it sucks and you don't want to believe it, but it's the truth.

Oh sure, there are stories out there of the wayward ex-wife crawling back to the husband, don't get me wrong. It happens. She may be tearful. She may be remorseful. She may be beyond regretful for the mistakes she made. She may do her absolute best to convince you, the betrayed man, that she learned from her mistakes and will never do those bad things ever again for as long as you both shall live. She may believe every single word of it.

She will be wrong, of course. Either consciously or unconsciously... she's lying about her future with you. She will either still be continuing on with her cheating in a more secretive way (rarely do they break contact completely with their affair partner), or she will just start all over again with somebody else in the near future. How do I know? Because I've seen this scenario played out hundreds of times, and I've never seen reconciliation work after discovering female infidelity. Never. Why? **Because your wife is now an addict.** Your wife is now an affair junky. She just got a taste of the high that only a new sexual relationship can offer. She just took a potent shot of sexual heroin. There's no going back now. No other drug on the planet compares to the thrill of a new lover. Your long-term comfortable relationship can't hold a candle to the feelings that a secret affair can bring about. Even the love for her own kids doesn't compare to the overwhelming nature of an affair. These new feelings of hers are a completely different ballgame.

Unfortunately, like all other addicts, she has to hit rock bottom before she sees the light and MAYBE gets better (this usually coincides with multiple failed affairs and her advancing age). You don't want to be around for rock bottom, trust me. Broken women usually take their man and everyone else down with them. It's not a pretty picture.

Let the relationship die. It's for the better. You will be okay. You have to trust me.

So, why did this happen to YOU? Well, that's the million dollar question every betrayed man wants the answer to, isn't it? WHAT could he have done to prevent it? WHY on Earth did his wife cheat on him? HOW did she lose feelings for him? HOW can

18

she just forget all they have done together over all these years? HOW can she so easily discard him like this? Is this just how it is with most women after so many years of marriage?

Why do we stress ourselves out with these questions over and over in our mind? Well, it's a perfectly natural part of the common grieving process for men. If you want to shoehorn it into the five common stages of grief (denial, anger, bargaining, depression and acceptance), it would probably fall under the "bargaining" category. It's a way for men to digest the trauma and eventually come to terms with the reality of the situation. For most men who have discovered an affair, there's an intense period of trying to make everything go back to the way it was before. Men are fixers, after all. We HAVE to figure out how and why the relationship machine broke down so suddenly, and what we can do to repair it and prevent it from ever happening again.

Contrary to what many men will tell you, the overall reason for the wife's affair and subsequent divorce is not as simple as, *"She's just a whore. All women are."* Sure, there are a ton of websites, forums, articles and angry male friends out there that will quickly use the *"all women are like that"* (AWALT) excuse as the explanation for what seems to be an epidemic of cheating wife behavior. Creating such a convenient excuse is a nice and simple way for you to place your anger at the feet of the opposite gender. You can wipe your hands of any and all responsibility and stop digging any further for the truth. It also feels nice to stick the proverbial knife deep into the person that hurt you so badly. What better way to hurt them then to say that they are just inherently EVIL and FLAWED to the core? They're cursed because they are a WOMAN and there's nothing she can do to stop being so awful.

So, what's the complete truth? Well, like most things in life… it's a little more complicated than you might think.

The reality is you had about a 50% shot of finding a wife that would stick by you for life and never divorce you. It's the flip of a coin. How about the chance that your wife will never have sexual desire for other men during your marriage? About 0%. She's a human being, after all. She has sexual needs just like you do. You want to have sex with others, right? Don't kid yourself. You watch porn and fantasize on a regular basis. It's perfectly okay to do so. Marrying somebody doesn't change your biology.

What were the chances of your wife acting on those natural desires and blowing up your life for the opportunity to sleep with other men? Well, that actually depends on a variety of factors, some of which are your responsibility as her partner.

We're human beings, so we like to think that when compared to our more primitive animal cousins, we have a stronger sense of right and wrong. We feel that we are somewhat immune to nature and all the urges and instincts we see our animal cousins acting out again and again. It's somewhat true, but not completely. Not understanding the full gamut of our surprisingly simple animalistic human nature is both naive and dangerous.

Human behavior is actually pretty damn predictable. In fact, we have an entire segment of the business world that is devoted to knowing the effective methods of pushing your psychological buttons in order to get you to act out in a certain way. We call it "marketing". Marketing uses a combination of visual, aural and psychological tricks to get you to take the necessary steps that will put you in the headspace to BUY something you most likely do not need. See, you have a *"make a spontaneous purchase"* button in your brain (the same button is also responsible for other impulsive behaviors like gambling, drugs, and overeating). Through the fascinating science of marketing, businesses slowly but surely push that button down just a little bit at a time. It may take seeing the product on Instagram and Facebook a few times, hearing about it on your favorite podcast a few times, seeing an ad for it during Monday Night Football, seeing your favorite Youtuber using the product, and hearing a few of your friends talk about the product…

but the button is eventually fully pressed down and you will find yourself at the point of purchase forking over your hard-earned cash (or, most likely, your credit card).

That buying decision was not random. It was no fluke. That was the result of a calculated plan by the advertiser and the product maker. Oh, don't feel too bad for buying that pointless widget. Plenty of people react in the exact same way. That's why the maker of the product you just bought has fifteen high-rise offices in three different countries, two factories, a fleet of private jets, and a company CEO that took home $32 million in bonuses last year. You're not alone in your impulsive purchasing decision. These impulses line the pockets of businessmen and keep our consumption-based economy humming along year after year.

You can take that same button-pushing marketing philosophy and apply it to other facets of human nature, like our mating habits. In the business world, you can use trial and error and an understanding of human psychology to come up with a plan and forecasts that show how much of the product X you believe you will sell, and how much money it will take to get to that goal. In the relationship world, the steps necessary to get a woman to cross the proverbial line into *"inappropriate behavior"* territory are just as predictable and quantifiable.

I have literally read hundreds of stories from men in your shoes. Are there obvious patterns to these stories? Oh, hell yes. All the stories are not exactly the same, but certain key points are so similar that I have compiled a list of items that need to take place to get your wife in the headspace necessary to cross the line, detach from you, and possibly have an affair.

1. Marriage

This one probably surprises you. Yes, if you want to increase the chances of your partner detaching from you and seeking out other sexual partners, then you should marry her. Allow me to explain.

We all know the tried-and-true trope of the girlfriend who had a wild and crazy sex drive prior to marriage, but she became a cold and timid shrew immediately after saying "I do". A lot of men in this state of marital hell believe that their wife committed a fraudulent "bait and switch" on them, trapping him and his resources with the implied promise of fantastic lifelong sex. The theory is that once her man shows his full commitment by taking her hand in marriage, she is then free to relax and show her TRUE asexual colors. *"I'm sorry. Sex is just not that important to me. Most women are like that."* she will often say.

Is this scenario really that common? Yes. Is it a matter of women just pretending to like sex up until the point of marriage, and then relaxing and ending the sexual charade once the ring goes on? Well, I'm sure that happens occasionally… but it's not as common as you think. There may be something else going on here.

"Familiarity breeds contempt." You've heard that one before, right? Usually interpreted as, *"When I see you every damn day, you start to annoy me, and I eventually dislike you."* As far as the woman in your life is concerned, it's more complex than that. The full story requires that you better understand the interesting but somewhat confounding world of the female mind.

Women want what they can't have. More specifically, if the relationship is a comfortable for-sure *"he's not going anywhere no matter what"* kind of relationship… then the process of shutting down the female sexual engine begins. For some women, the simple act of marriage can shut off the desire for her man completely. She won the prize, now she doesn't want it anymore. It's that little bit of early relationship anxiety and insecurity she used to have that started the process of pushing her *"Must have sex with this man"* button. You can think of it as mother nature telling her, *"This man must be important and desired by many women if he's not eager to immediately settle down with you. Is he seeing other girls!? If so, he must be a really valuable mate! You should make a baby with him while you have the chance! Lock him down!"*

She needs that excitement. She needs that uncertainty. She needs that newness and spontaneity. When she locks you down, you become a *"for sure"* thing. You're not going anywhere. That *"must have sex with my man"* button is just not pushed down as much as it used to be. Over time the button pushed down less and less... and eventually, cobwebs start to form around it.

Keep in mind that the comfort of marriage can very well shut down the libido of the wife... but not necessarily for every man on the planet and for every situation. Her libido is by no means turned off completely, as most men seem to think. Women can be extremely horny creatures, but just not always for their husbands. That is a fact many men seem completely blind to, even after watching their wives stare at man butts, read erotic novels (Fifty Shades of Grey made bazillions in book and movie sales), and listen to her talk to her friends about the cute guy at the office. Her brain is most definitely in "scan for new man meat" mode while married (just like you enjoy staring at pretty women). **The ugly truth is that, for many women, the comfort and familiarity of marriage take her husband out of that long list of guys she would gladly have wild and crazy sex with.**

The grand irony of marriage: **Women want to get married.** Women want the big wedding. They want the house and 2.5 kids. They want the white picket fence, the dog and the doting husband that helps out with the child-rearing and the housework. They absolutely positively genuinely want all of that. It's their lifelong dream. Unfortunately, their primitive sex drive disagrees. Inside their brain, there is a battle going on between their social conditioning, their need for safety and security, and the DNA that encapsulates hundreds of thousands of years of female reproductive strategy and instinct telling her to keep her options open. Instinct often wins if the environment is just right.

23

CHAPTER 1: WHY DID THIS HAPPEN?

2. Stress

There's early relationship anxiety, and then there's the stress and pressure of real everyday life. These are two totally different things for the female libido. The stress and insecurity of everyday life absolutely kill a woman's sex drive for her husband. The further you remove her from the fantasy world of the lustful beginnings of the hot and heavy relationship, the more her sex drive withers away. Yet, it's important to remember that with stress and the declining sex drive at home comes the opposite effect outside of the home. Your wife has human needs and they're not being met. Her body and brain know this. In fact, the stress of life makes her NEED for excitement and escape from her life grow exponentially. This is why the most affair-prone person in a relationship is the professional working mom who has way too much on her plate. Her affair button is in a constant state of being almost pushed all the way down, and it doesn't take much at all to press it fully and for her to cross the line in a really bad way.

Let me illustrate further the difference between men and women and the relationship between sex drive and stress. Think about a really shitty and stressful day at work. Your boss calls you into his office to let you know that the company will be making some cuts to the staff. He may have to let you go. It's not 100% sure yet. He's trying to convince the big bosses to keep you and your team on the job, but it's not looking good. He wanted to let you know so that you can prepare in case he does have to fire all of you. Now you're in an ultra-stressed state of employment limbo. *"Will I get fired? Do I get a paycheck next month? What will my wife think?"*

If after this news you went home and told your wife all the horrible details of your day and she said, *"Alright... you know what you need, mister? You need a blowjob"*, you would be all for it. No questions asked. Hallelujah. A blowjob is absolutely the best medicine at that moment. Your "ready for sex" button is always at the edge of being fully pressed down, and hearing *"Blowjob?"* pushes it the rest of the way. At that moment you feel like you have the best wife on the planet Earth. With that one act, she just validated you and your worth as a man.

Let's look at this scenario in a much more realistic way. The husband comes home and says to the wife, *"We need to talk."* He then dumps on her all of this horrible news about the meeting with his boss and his job possibly going away. Instantly, the wife starts thinking about bills not being paid, the lights getting turned off, not being able to care for the kids properly, not buying stuff she wants when she wants, her friends finding out that her husband is unemployed… It's all too much to bear.

Sex with her husband? A blowjob? What about it?! Uh, no thank you! Her sex drive is now completely shut down. Sex with her husband is not even an option when life dumps such a stressful load of shit in her lap. Her body and brain just said to her, *"The Provider male is no longer able to care for you and the family. He can't protect you. Shut down the sexual engine immediately. You don't want to have a baby with this horrible financial situation hanging over your head. This male is a suboptimal life mate."* In relatively short time, her body and brain may very well say, *"Time to look at alternative mates that can better provide for us."* It's not evil, as some would contend. It's human nature.

"So, let me get this straight" men all say. *"She's turned off by the comfort and familiarity of married life, and she's turned off when shit hits the fan and life gets stressful for her? Both comfort and stress within the marriage cause her to shut down sexually?"* Yes, exactly. *"So, we can't win!"* No, you can, but most men don't have the relationship skills needed to acquire and KEEP a loyal wife through all of life's hard times. It's tremendously hard to maintain a long-lasting, romantic relationship with a woman. More on that in chapter three, *"Succeeding in Relationships"*.

25

3. Loss of Respect

This one sure does upset a lot of men. Simply put, if your wife loses respect for you, she's certainly not turned on by you. As soon as she deems you unworthy of her respect, she will immediately have her eyes open and scanning for Mr. Replacement (this may or may not be a conscious decision on her part). Do you know how many times I've heard from men that have been dumped by their partner, *"Well, my wife got a promotion at work and she started making a lot more than me"* or, *"I was laid off from work and couldn't find a job for 3 months, but that was okay because her job was more than enough to pay the bills for a while"*? It is very common. For some women, the mere idea of their man making less money than them is enough to dry up their marital sex drive and start the process of emotionally detaching. Yes, it's stupid and shallow, but it's certainly not unheard of.

This need for respect is so strong, that sometimes money isn't the issue, but the PERCEPTION of money and status is. For example, I had a guy contact me who made way more money than his wife. She worked at a big corporation in some pointless management job, sitting at a cubicle making five figures a year doing pointless cost-saving projects. He, on the other hand, made six figures by working several different productive jobs at once. He owned and managed several rental properties, ran a small landscaping company with his brother, and sold collectibles on eBay. It wasn't a "traditional" one paycheck job, but it was honest work, gave his family plenty of money, and…. he was happy! The wife, though… she was obviously not too impressed. She often pestered him about applying for a job at her company.

Him: "Why would I stop what I'm doing now to go work in an office and make just $60k like you? I make way more than that."

Her: "Well, you'd have more job security, for one thing."

Him: "Your company just laid off a bunch of people last year. Remember how you were all stressed about it? How is that more security?"

Her: "Well, I just don't think you should shut out opportunities like this. A lot of people would kill for a job there."

This topic started coming up ALL the time. He finally figured out what the real problem was. He noticed when they were at company gatherings or meeting people for the first time, his wife would get really weird when people asked him what he did for a living. She always tried to change the topic or walked away from the conversation. He eventually asked her about it and she admitted that, yes, it was kind of embarrassing to hear him tell people he was a landlord, landscaper and eBay seller. Other husbands in their group had normal jobs like a Dentist or Sales Manager. It made him sound like a loser in comparison. She didn't want to be seen as the wife of a loser.

He was completely insulted and shocked by her admission. The woman he loved was telling him this shallow nonsense. The mother of his children. His best friend. Did she forget that he brought home way more money than she did?! Did she forget all the things he has paid for over the years? Also, he was no dummy. He was an educated man. He was intelligent. He was hard-working. He busted his butt every single day for the family… and he was extremely happy while doing it. To him, that was a win-win. To his wife, all that mattered was that his perceived value was possibly low in comparison to other men. She was afraid of what her social group may think.

This lack of respect was eventually the straw that broke the camel's back, and it wasn't long before she finally filed for divorce.

She did so after jumping on a man with a suitable job title and social cache. **It's common knowledge that women rarely leave a relationship without having another one standing by.**

His lack of a "good enough" job title wasn't THE thing that ruined their marriage. In hindsight, his marriage troubles began shortly after his wife had their third kid. He saw numerous red flags that showed she wasn't coping well with the changing relationship dynamics and the stress that came with being a working parent of three. Her pressuring him to take on a different job was just a last-ditch effort to keep the marital machine running. *"Please, at least change your job so I can have some respect for you and possibly stop these repeated feelings I have about leaving you."*

This one stings for a lot of guys because it cuts to the heart of the matter and exposes the ugly side of the relationship. It shows that his wife's love for him does, in fact, have conditions, and one of the conditions may be as simple as stupid as, *"Have a job title that impresses my social group"*. The good husband is proud to say he sticks with his wife through thick and thin, loves her for her mind and her heart, overlooked things like her weight gain and often bitchy attitude, is proud to call her his wife... but she started to look for a replacement because his job title or paycheck was not that impressive?! Yes. It happens.

4. She Becomes Your Mother

Parenthood and sexual desire do not work in tandem; they work against each other. Being a parent is the antithesis of being a sexual human being. When your wife is in mom mode, she's only in mom mode. When the baby is screaming, the 12-year-old is saying he's hungry again, the dog just knocked over his water bowl, and she has a washer full of mildewy laundry she forgot to put in the dryer the night before... the last thing she wants is for her needy/horny husband to come behind her and poke her in the butt with his erection. He may see it as a sexy joke, but his wife sees it as a show of disrespect and lack of awareness of the awful situation spinning around in her brain. The husband might as well take a giant shit on her head. Same result. It just adds to the chaos.

If you REALLY want to take your wife out of the sexy headspace, then become her adult child. Become completely dependent upon her for your day-to-day living. Add to the stressful chaos of her life. Become part of the problem and not a solution. Make sure that she is the only one to organize and make things happen in the family. She makes your dentist appointments, she tells you what clothes to wear to special events, she tells you when you're going out to see your couple friends, she cleans up after you, she feeds you, etc. All of this is not a good recipe for the female libido. You're just another mouth to feed. Another butt to wipe. You're a helpless creature. Respect goes right out the window with such behavior. She desperately NEEDS you to take charge on occasion and show her your independence. Show her that you can absolutely positively be a happy and productive person if you had to live on your own. A woman that rolls her eyes and laughs at the thought of her helpless husband living alone is a woman who wants nothing to do with him sexually. *"Oh, God. I can't imagine Robert on his own. He would probably die of starvation or drown in dirty laundry. He's helpless."*

Now, this doesn't mean that running around and doing chores gets your wife turned on and ready for sex and happily committed to you for life. You don't do household chores to win the favor of your wife and "get lucky" (that's called "chore play"). You do these things because you're an adult and they need to get done. Whatever you do, don't you dare do the dishes and then sulk when she doesn't want to give you a blowjob that night. Children run to mommy to show her that they cleaned up messes and hope for hugs and a *"GOOD JOB!!"*. You never want to find yourself saying, *"Honey, I washed the dishes and did laundry!"* Oh, wow. What do you want, a cookie? No, you want love and affection from your wife.

29

It's obvious and it's a complete turnoff. It just sets off her brain's *"This man is not worthy of my respect and time"* response.

5. Other Women Lost Interest in You, and You Lost Interest in Other Women

This one is a real head-scratcher for a lot of guys. Many wives will punish and shame their husbands if he is to look at or make any kind of sexual reference to other women. The husband says, *"Oh, she's cute"*, and the wife immediately stops what she's doing and scowls. *"Cute!? How can you think that's a good thing to say? She's like 20 years old. Do you like teen girls, too? What about your daughter's friends? You should really think before you say stuff like that because it's creepy and hurtful to me."* Ouch. Husband goes back to his man cave with his tail between his legs. The message is clear: No other girls are attractive. Ever. Only his wife. To think otherwise is sacrilege.

The wife's shaming of her husband's sexuality is an extremely common scenario. It's kind of an understood cultural norm. This is why men have always hidden their porn, sneak away to strips clubs with their buddies, and look straight down at their shoes when that curvy brunette walks by them in the mall. Even the most basic and innocent of actions can set off the wife, and most men can't deal with the stress of a hostile wife. Men just want peace and quiet.

The irony (and there's a lot of irony in relationships, as you'll learn) is that much of this "flirty" or "eye wandering" behavior that wives shame their husbands for is a crucial piece to unlocking the combination to the wife's own sexual needs. Simply put, a man that has sexual options in life is a total turn-on (if you're 500 lbs. and unemployed, this does not pertain to you). If your woman can drop you off at any random bar on a Friday night and never has to worry about women coming on to you, then you are NOT a turn-on. You are a comfortable life partner. You are a for-sure thing. Remember,

comfort and boredom kill the female libido. There needs to be that little bit of uncertainty to keep the flame going. It's one thing to be a good, faithful husband. It's another thing to be a neutered man shamed into pretending to not have urges that every other man on the planet has… just so you don't piss off your wife.

For a married woman, one of the absolute biggest turn-ons is to go to a social event with her man and watch other people, especially women, admire him. If a pretty woman goes up to her man and chats and makes flirty eyes at him, and her husband reciprocates, that's a man that is going home that night and getting laid by his wife. Her man went from normal everyday husband to the guy that other high-value women find attractive. His sexual ranking just went through the roof in one night… and all he did was stand there and be himself. He put in zero work, and mother nature rewarded him. That's a man that stands above the crowd. That's a man who has a wife who says, *"I'm really really lucky to have a man like THAT."*

Get married, stress your wife out, have her lose respect for you, make yourself completely unattractive, and don't think about other women… so, that's it? That's the secret combination for triggering female infidelity? Yes, it seems to be for many women. *"Well, whatever happened to being faithful!?"* I hear that a lot from guys. Let's be honest, not all women will reach the point of actually pulling the trigger on an affair. Some will just accept a blah dead bedroom marriage while living a wild fantasy life of romance novels and the occasional rough pornography. Some bored women may even go as far as taking control of their marital sex life and do what they can to reignite the fire themselves (this is super rare).

Yes, all women have the capacity to cheat. Just like you do. Just like I do. We're human beings, after all. I would hope that the life experiences that led you to buy this book have shown you what women are completely capable of. They don't belong on the pedestal

31

of perfection you probably put them on. They're no better and no worse than you.

As human beings, women have one particular truism that rings true for both sexes: **Show me their childhood, and I'll show you their future.**

Borderline Personality Disorder

There is a particular circumstance in the life of women that seems to the lay the groundwork for possible mental illness and future relationship trouble: **abandonment by a parent.** This could be dad leaving, mom leaving, mom and dad divorcing, etc. The commonality in all of these situations is that the child perceived a life of love and security, and it was suddenly yanked away from them. Their little malleable brains aren't wired to deal with the trauma of living in an uncertain world with a missing parental figure. We know now that the number one predictor of Borderline Personality Disorder (BPD) in women is abandonment. Mom or dad left her when she was young, and she's "acting out" this trauma on all of her subsequent relationship partners for the rest of her life. Some men like to call it severe "daddy issues". Whatever you want to call it, it's yet another example of our predictable human behavior.

BPD is the extreme form of "broken woman" that is, unfortunately, becoming more and more common. Take a woman from a broken home who has never been taught coping skills or boundaries of any kind, and you have a good chance that she develops full-blown BPD. Not every woman who was abandoned has BPD, but every woman with BPD was abandoned.

Here are the common BPD behaviors. See if these ring any bells.

1. Love bombing.
When that initial infatuation/falling in love/"I must

procreate with this man" stage hits, it hits the BPD woman hard. Really hard. She will do anything and everything to be with her new man. She will shower him with praise. She will buy him things. She will submit to any and all sexual needs the man may have. She will lose weight. She will dress seductively. She will text or call incessantly. The sex will be amazing. For a man with little dating experience and/or feelings of low self-esteem, this is absolutely the most amazing feeling he has ever experienced. This HAS to mean she is "the one" for him, right?!

"I just knew she was the one from the first day we met." I've heard this more than a few times from my readers who have BPD wives. The worshipping of the BPD partner by the low self-worth man starts right away.

Let's be honest. All men want a woman who love bombs them. To be worshipped and adored at such an extreme level (by such a beautiful and sexual creature) is our dream. Oh, to be king for a day! When we are in the midst of experiencing an extreme BPD love bomb, what should be obvious warning signs of way-too-early and extreme attachment are drowned out by all the fantastic positive emotions we men feel (and the fantastic porn sex, of course).

"When wearing rose-colored glasses, all the red flags just look like flags."

2. Extreme Jealousy

The BPD woman is extremely threatened by the emotional connections you make with others. This could be your attachment to your children, your coworkers, your platonic friends, your ex-girlfriends, etc. She will do all she can to separate you physically and emotionally from these people. In her mind, she must eliminate all competition for her attention.

Her brain: *"Stop all these other relationships! He's going to leave you!"*

3. Morphing

Women are naturally more agreeable and pliable than men. We all know the woman who takes on the personality traits, hobbies, and interests of her new boyfriend. She didn't use to like football, now all of a sudden, she's wearing a Bengals jersey and yelling at the TV during Monday Night Football.

The BPD woman takes this to the next level. She doesn't have that filter or boundary mechanism that says, *"Oh, I like you and all… but I'm not doing THAT. I have self-respect."* Instead, she will gladly put on the football jersey, snort the cocaine, pop the pills, get the tattoo, get the boob job, join the orgy, and ignore her kids for weeks at a time. This is all in an effort to keep the new man around and avoid the abandonment she fears more than anything.

4. Splitting.

What was once the best thing in the entire universe is now the equivalent of dog shit on the bottom of her shoe. This sudden change in thought, or "splitting", can seem to happen suddenly with no warning. Then, the dog shit goes back to being fantastic again… but only briefly. Then it's back to being awful again. Usually that piece of dog shit is the unsuspecting male partner in her life. The husband or boyfriend she was once infatuated with becomes a laughable loser when she meets and bonds with a new man.

Again, this is common cheating woman behavior. Where the BPD woman takes it a step further is that she goes WAY BEYOND indifference towards her ex and has to actively try to destroy him. She will reach out to her social circle to ruin his name. She may try to physically harm him or get others to do it. She may take all his money. She will randomly send him messages reminding him of just how worthless he is. She will tell the kids how awful he is. She will outright lie about him to anyone he cares about.

She won't stop until he is completely destroyed.

She's getting back at him for "abandoning" her. It doesn't matter that SHE cheated and broke up with him and attached to another man. In her reptilian brain, she was abandoned by her ex. He failed to play the role she needed. He must pay the price.

There is no grey area with a BPD woman. It's all or nothing. **You're either the second coming of Jesus or the Devil himself.**

The "Oh wow, this is really fucked up" moment comes when the abused man finally gets wise and decides to stop all contact with the BPD woman. That is when she is left with her acute fear of abandonment. This is when she will lash out in more anger, sadness and may even self-harm or attempt suicide. This draws the ex back in… and then the cycle continues.

5. Gaslighting

This is a term used when abusive people try to convince you that the red flags you are seeing are actually YOUR fault. YOU'RE the crazy/mean/cruel/abusive one. She's the victim.

With the BPD woman, it is never her fault. It never will be her fault. She can't see the rational side of things because she is incapable of doing so.

This just makes the "nice guy" husband want to try even harder. After all, he made vows to this woman. For better or for worse. Maybe she has a point. That one time he did say she was acting like a bitch… he shouldn't have done that. He can be a better husband. She sees his groveling and his attempts to fix the situation, and she grows more resentful and angrier.

This form of abuse has lasting repercussions for the man and his subsequent relationships moving forward in life. He questions everything about himself and his already low self-esteem is completely flushed down the toilet.

"Maybe I AM the problem. Maybe I'm worthless."

6. Infidelity
In broad terms, BPD women feel two things:

1. An intense need for love and acceptance.
2. A need to engage in impulsive and risky behavior to elicit a feeling of being "alive".

Cheating fits in perfectly with their psyche.

You, the nice/normal guy with low self-esteem, will never be enough for the BPD woman. NOBODY will be enough for her. This is the ultimate irony of BPD. She is frightened to the core about the chance of abandonment by her partner, but she does everything in her power to drive him away… including abuse and actually running into the arms of another man (or multiple men). A BPD woman will often rationalize her frequent infidelities by saying, *"Hey, we all know you were going to cheat on me, anyway."*

Yes, "normal" women cheat all the time. The BPD difference is that they often like to rub it in the face of the ex-partner. There are stories of women sending photos of them engaging in sex with their new man, sharing graphic details, explaining how the new partner is physically better/more endowed, etc. This is just part of the *"must punish the old partner for not doing what he was supposed to"* pathology. Whatever she can do to chip away at the confidence and happiness of the ex-partner, she will do.

Baggage

When men tell me about their ex going crazy and leaving him and the kids to go run off with some loser guy with a face tattoo, the first words out of my mouth are usually: *"So, tell me about her mom."* Invariably, I will hear horror stories about their wife's crazy narcissistic mom who spent years jumping from man to man, had a history of substance abuse, frequently abandoned her kids, often got fired from a list of menial jobs, etc. Mom was a real mess… and she was probably the wife's number one female role model in life. That role model did not provide the sanity and security she needed while growing up. She provided the exact opposite. I've heard this more than a few times: *"It's funny. She always despised everything her mom stood for. Couldn't stand her. Then she became an exact carbon copy of her."*

Popular culture likes to demonize the "deadbeat dad"; the guy who walked away from his family and refuses to help provide for the children. Yes, that scenario does exist. These stereotypes don't fall from the sky, after all. Men are completely capable of being awful humans, as we are all well aware of. But, what we don't often hear about is the toxic mom. While the absent father may plant seeds of abandonment in the sensitive and malleable child's brain, it's the toxic mom that will further poison them and continuously feed their brains a steady diet of awfulness that will have repercussions for the rest of their life. In short, was her mom a basket case? Then your wife's capacity for being the same is very high.

Your ex's childhood is a big part of what we call her personal "baggage". Baggage is another word for all the negative stuff that happened to her in the past and is now deeply embedded in her psyche and ready to bubble up at a moment's notice. So, when your wife starts acting crazy and rebellious and has abandoned the kids, she's probably acting out all the psychological baggage in her life that she never properly dealt with. He mom did crazy stuff when she was a kid… she never properly processed or got help with how to deal with it… and she becomes her mom. Simple. It's textbook behavior.

To further illustrate the concept, picture baggage as a bunch of luggage in the back of a car. A woman who has a shit ton of baggage is barreling down the road in a car with suitcases and duffle bags poking out of the back windows. The trunk is so full that it can't close. It's stuck open and tied down with bungee cords. It's a mess. The weight of the baggage is so much that it actually throws off the balance of the car. She has to keep her hands on the wheel at all times and constantly make corrections with little tugs left and right. The second she takes her hands off the wheel… SCREEECH! She's off the road and headed for a tree. Disaster.

A person's baggage will absolutely have a negative impact on their life and their relationships with others… unless they recognize the baggage for what it is, live in reality, and take steps towards remedying the situation. Unfortunately, for many women, they have been fed a steady diet of *"you are perfect the way you are"* and *"you go girl"* throughout their long history of poor life decisions. She has a growing fan club of friends and family ready to applaud her every step of the way. The thought of being "damaged" and needing to do the hard work to improve themselves is pushed aside in favor of living in the moment and in a fog of artificial happiness that everyone in their life seems to glorify.

Now, men, I'm not about to let you off the hook. You have your own baggage you never dealt with, too. I'm just going by the dozens of guys I've spoken to over the years, and it's safe to say that they all had baggage that helped lead them to the awful situation they found themselves in. They all had childhood issues they never quite dealt with effectively, and it bit them on the ass in the worst way. For most of these guys, they had a series of life events that eventually gave them a bad case of Nice Guy Syndrome.

Nice Guy Syndrome

After reading this book, I whole-heartedly recommend you go out and buy a copy of **"No More Mr. Nice Guy"** by Dr. Robert Glover. I have recommended that book to hundreds of guys over the years, and all who bought it came back to me and said it was the ultimate eye-opener for them.

Dr. Glover has done an excellent job of identifying and helping to eliminate a phenomenon that has brought down so many men. I won't go into all the specifics of the book, but the core tenant is that so many of us men have been led to believe that we should be as agreeable as possible and not rock the boat when it comes to our interpersonal relationships. As a result, people in our lives (women in particular) will walk all over us. This makes us bitter and not-so-nice men that live in a world of what we feel SHOULD be rather than what IS. We get mad when people who we have personal relationships with don't act in the particular way that we expect them to… but, we never tell these people exactly what it is we expect of them! This is what Dr. Glover calls a *"covert contract"*.

Here's a very real-world example of a covert contract in action:

Your wife tells you that she is going out with her friends from work next Friday. They're all celebrating a coworker's birthday. Amongst the group of friends planning to go out is an ex-boyfriend of your wife. Understandably, you don't feel exactly right about it, but you don't feel comfortable telling your wife how you really feel. For one thing, you don't want to come across as a jealous, controlling husband. After all, your wife SHOULD know better than to go out partying with an ex-boyfriend. You shouldn't HAVE to tell her. Plus, you don't have the energy to deal with the possible drama that will erupt from you saying NO to her. So, you tell her you don't mind at all and decide to sit back and watch what she does. As planned, she goes out with the friends (and the ex-

39

boyfriend) for a wild night of drinking.

Your wife drunkenly texts you throughout the night. Each text gets a little sillier and more nonsensical. You're trying to read the kids a bedtime story, and she's happily texting things like, *"OMG. Stacey just spilled her drink on Sally's crotch! She looks like she peed her pants!! LOL!"* After a few more of those messages, you are officially beyond annoyed. You are seething and barely able to sleep. She eventually returns home and stumbles into bed after 3:00 am.

The next morning, she is badly hung over and not able to help out with the kids and their normal Saturday morning routine. She just lays in bed moaning and saying she feels like she's going to throw up. The more she whines, the angrier you get. You go online and see her social media posts with images from the night before. There are dozens of photos of them hanging out at the bar getting drunker and drunker as the night goes on. Lots of laughing and dancing. There are exactly twelves photos of her with her ex-boyfriend. They are posing together for the camera, joking around and making drunken sexual poses with each other. One of the photos makes it look like he is humping her doggy style while she grabs her friend's boobs... in a fully-clothed pseudo threesome. Hilarious. They're laughing and spilling their drinks, having a great time. You're officially livid. THIS is not the behavior of a mom or of a wife. This is completely embarrassing and inappropriate.

You start stomping around the house, picking up messes and doing household chores, grunting and loudly sighing with every movement. Your wife finally sits up in bed and asks, *"What's wrong with you?"* That's it. You can't hold back anymore. *"What's wrong with ME?! What's wrong with YOU? What kind of mom goes out drinking and partying with an ex-boyfriend until 3:00 am!? Those photos you posted online are fucking embarrassing! You're a married mom of two kids! What is wrong with you?!"* The wife is shocked. Instead of apologizing, she points the finger right back at you. *"I told you what we had planned. I asked you if it was ok. Obviously, you had a real problem with it. Why didn't you just tell me you didn't want me to go? I would've stayed home. I didn't HAVE to go. It was just innocent fun with the old gang from work."* How does every nice guy husband respond in this scenario? *"I shouldn't HAVE to tell you!"*

In this example, both the husband and wife do have a valid point, but the responsibility for how the whole situation played out ultimately lays at the feet of the husband. He was asked for his opinion up front, and he didn't have the balls to share his true feelings. He chickened out. He didn't want to rock the boat. He didn't want to come across as a controlling asshole. In a roundabout way, he was actually being MORE controlling in the end. He knew exactly how that night would turn out, and he held back his opinion just so he could later have his *"Ah ha! Gotcha!"* moment. He'll never admit it, but it was a passive aggressive stunt. Most nice guys are experts at passive aggressiveness and holding back their true feelings at the right moment.

The nice guy won't dare tell his wife that she needs to eat better and lose weight. He won't tell his wife when she's acting like a bitch. He won't tell the boss at work that he deserves a raise. He won't tell his friends that he expects them to help him move to his new apartment, especially since he helped them so many times. Instead, he will just sit back, watch the people in his life act against his best interests... and he will be pissed about it. He feels they should all be acting better and more aware of his feelings. The resentment builds and builds until he eventually blows his top or just quietly lives a life of stress and regret.

The nice guy introduces stress and resentment into his life (and subsequently into the lives of those around him) simply because he refuses to play the part of the bad guy for a few measly seconds. The man with the rapidly expanding wife should've sat her down and told her that he loves her with all his heart, but looks and health are very important to him, and they should be important to her, too. Starting tomorrow they will start working out together so she can lose weight and be a woman he is attracted to and a good healthy role model for the kids. The man being pushed around at work and being passed over for a promotion should tell his boss that he has worked his butt off for so many years and brings a lot of value to the company and therefore deserves a raise. The man with the asshole friends should tell them that he has always been there for them when they needed him the most and he expects them to drop what they're doing every now and then to help when he needs them, too. These are things that men with a strong sense of self-worth do. This is a mentally healthy approach to life and conflict in general.

The commonality in all of these honest dude moments is the recognition that he is taking a risk by standing up for himself. He's more than willing to take the loss if he has to. The husband is willing to divorce a lazy overweight wife who just doesn't care anymore, the employee is polishing his resume and ready to resign at any moment, and the annoyed guy is willing to tell his deadbeat friends to fuck off. In other words, a strong man realizes that he needs to stand up for himself and his principles… but he knows that it may not end the way he wants it to. He's prepared for that. The honest man knows that if he just tries to smooth things over and be the nice guy all the time, it will just make matters worse. Being nice all the time is just a form of denial.

Being nice is also another way of saying that you are being a very agreeable person. Agreeableness is one of the big five personality traits and it is most common in women. When you just go with the flow and don't put your foot down and stick up for yourself, you're being more effeminate and therefore more unattractive to women who are looking for the opposite.

Putting Women on a Pedestal

A man notices that his wife has been acting strangely over the past couple of months. She's been putting in way more hours at work. She's been going out regularly with her friends. She has been dressing sexier and lost a lot of weight. She's been on her phone non-stop. She will often bicker and snap at her husband for no apparent reason, seemingly trying to start fights on a daily basis. He saw her texting somebody and then deleting the texts when he walked by. Weird.

The husband is talking to a friend over beers and he brings up his wife's strange behavior. His friend listens and grows more concerned with every detail of the story. Finally, his friend stops him and says, *"Wait. Dude. Come on. Seriously? She's totally cheating on you."* Husband is taken aback by this accusation. *"What?! No, dude. She's not like that. She's very much against cheating. Always has been. It's gotta be something else."*

Men just love to put their women up on the pedestal of moral perfection. Even with mounting evidence of wrongdoing, a man will often be in complete denial, unable to see what is so obvious to everyone around him. *"Nope, not my wife. No way."* Even after discovering that she is lying to him, he will quickly let that slide. *"Okay, she lied about THAT... but she would never do that OTHER thing."* He keeps moving the goalposts. He keeps changing the rules so that she never wins the coveted *"She's just a broken, awful human being after all"* trophy. To nice guys with no boundaries and a fear of conflict (and the possibility of abandonment), there is no choice but to put the woman at a higher moral level than him. She is the beacon of hope in a world filled with dread and anxiety. If that crumbles, what does he have left to lean on?

Why is it so common for men to put women on a pedestal? What is going on in the mind of a man that he would elevate a normal human to superhuman levels... just because of their gender? Well, like with most things in life, it starts when we are young. For a lot of men, a combination of puberty and childhood social anxiety caused girls to be highly desirable, but frustratingly off-limits. The boy's own fears, sexual shame, and low self-image put up unnatural barriers between themselves and girls. For high-anxiety/low self-esteem boys, there is nothing as terrifying as asking a girl out and possibly being rejected.

As we mature and become horny out-of-control late teen boys, the pedestalization gets further amplified. We are torn between feelings of romance/love and unbridled testosterone-fueled horniness. We dream of walking hand-in-hand with Ms. Perfect, talking on the phone for hours, going to the movies… and we also fantasize about banging her in the basement on the washing machine while the parents are gone. During the spin cycle, of course. Our shameful male sexuality is at odds with our need for female companionship. We've been told again and again to subdue our sexuality and to prop up our sweet and thoughtful behaviors instead. Being a *"gentleman"*, we are told, is key for *"winning"* the hand of a good girl. The common lingo of terms like *"winning"* and *"getting lucky"* are examples of social norms that serve to elevate the woman to superhuman levels and further shame the male for his natural inclinations. This all starts at very young age for all men.

After years of nice guy behavior and pedestalization of women in his life, the typical nice guy has an elaborate fantasy life where all the pretty girls in his social circle suddenly realize just how nice and perfect he is. No longer does he have to watch the good-looking jocks and confident assholes date the prettiest and sweetest girls in class. His sex life will then reach levels of awesome depravity only seen in the pornography he has become addicted to. Obviously, this is a fantasy that never pans out. He may say he's too much of a gentleman, not a dumb jock, too smart, or too kind, but the truth is that he's just too scared to make the obvious changes needed to become successful with women.

After finally landing a woman (usually she has to approach him or he is pushed to her by friends), the nice guy latches on like a tick and will not let go no matter what happens. This inevitably results in a man who gladly overlooks numerous red flags under the guise of being a sensitive and understanding partner. The entirety of his being is centered around the relationship with his woman. He has no choice but to overlook red flags. Without her and their relationship, he has nothing of real substance in his life. Everyone else in his social circle probably takes advantage of him in some way, so to come home to *"unconditional"* love from his perfect wife is an oasis in the desert of life's awfulness. To suddenly tell him that the oasis was really a mirage all along is traumatizing. *"Nope. She would never do that. She's not like that."*

Putting women on a pedestal is also a subtle form of sexism. Women are often looked at as timid, overly kind, weak little pixies of love and romance. They need to be handled gently or else they will spaz out uncontrollably in fits of emotion. As a result, many people think we can't involve women in such rational or tough-minded things such as running a business or playing a sport. We also can't involve them in the perverse male-centered world of our sexuality. They're women. They're way different. They're actually BETTER, in many ways, we tell ourselves. They belong up on the pedestal looking down on us sport-playing, porn-loving, penis-having ingrates.

It's all bullshit, of course. Not only is it demeaning to paint women with such a wide behavioral brush, but it's only setting men up for severe future relationship failure. A man sees the woman as a delicate creature worthy of praise and optimism... when he should be treating her with the same level of rational skepticism he applies to the men in his life. She's a human being. She can be an evil, sex-loving, business-running, violent asshole, too.

Not only is putting women on a pedestal unrealistic and

unfair, it is also a potent female libido killer. SHE wants to look up to HIM, not look down on him. If you put her up on the highest of pedestals, she has no choice but to look down on you… and thus lose respect for you. She may say she wants to be treated like a princess, but only if her man is a king. The nerd who brings flowers to the prom queen and professes his love will get turned down around 100% of the time. The tall handsome jock with a natural charm who hands the prom queen a half-eaten piece of beef jerky and says, *"Yer kinda hot, I guess"* will get laughs and lots of sex in the not-too-distant future.

Weakness and Vulnerability Are Not a Male Virtue

There has been much talk recently about *"toxic masculinity"*. The thought is that we, as men, have been held captive by a *"be a tough alpha male no matter what"* philosophy. This has led to an emotionally stunted population of men with mental health issues (such as a much higher suicide rate). Toxic Masculinity is also seen as being responsible for things such as war, rape, sexual assault and violence in general. The theory is that once we stomp out this evil toxic mindset (and allow for our more positive, sedate, thoughtful, feminine side to take hold), we will all be better off.

Yeah, no. It doesn't work that way. Sounds great on paper, doesn't pan out in real life.

Yes, it's true, most men have been taught at an early age to suck it up. To not emote too damn much. To remain stoic in the face of danger. We've been taught that the noblest of men will not run from danger, but actually run towards the danger and rescue and help those in need. The fireman runs into the burning building. The soldier runs into a hail of bullets to save the fallen comrade. The captain of the sinking ship boat yells, *"Women and children first!"* The message is simple: Be tough. Be strong. We need you, men. Without you, life is a dangerous, chaotic place. This is true

46

now more than ever… but the message is now getting drowned out by the incessant call for men to *"open up"* more and not play the part of the tough guy all the damn time.

The result? Well, ask any man who has displayed weakness to his woman. At first, she appreciates the vulnerability (*"He trusts me enough to let me in and see his weak side! I love it!"*), but only up to a point. There is a very real, and very quick switch where the sentiment goes from, *"This is normal human vulnerability I can appreciate and relate to"* to *"Ew… stop. Gross. What kind of man are you?"* If you've lived long enough and have had relationships with women, you've seen the switch flipped. Women can only tolerate so much weakness from the man they want so badly to lean on and look up to. They want a strong oak tree to depend on, not a frail little sapling still trying to find his emotional way in life.

The misconception is that *"toxic masculinity"* is pushed on us by our fellow men. The thought is that we men have informally gathered together as a group and decided to make life tough and as hard as possible on each other. *"Dave over there is crying! Quick, somebody slap him and call him gay! Point and laugh. That'll teach him."* The idea is preposterous. In fact, if you get a room of men, and only men, together for the sake of helping each other out (like a therapy group or rehab), you will see **a lot** of crying. Men feel safe opening up to other men they know and respect. You'll see men talk about love and life and hugging each other as all emotionally healthy people do. But, put a woman in that group and watch the tears dry up. The hugs will stop. No more *"I love you, man"*. No more talks about the time John was beaten or molested as a kid. Why? Because a woman is in the room. The woman rules the emotional relationship landscape. The message has been made clear to all men: **Respect is everything to women**. Want a relationship with a woman to last? Then you better be strong. You better win her respect. Women have shown us this for generations. We have listened. We have responded.

In a sense, women are the cause of *"toxic"* masculinity. The push for men to emote is, subconsciously, a giant test of a man's strength (**see more about female tests in chapter three "Succeeding in Relationships"**). Pass the test, win her respect and get the girl. This is a universal truth we have all taken to heart.

The Mysterious Female Sex Drive

One area that many men underestimate or completely misunderstand is the subject of female sexual desire. Most men assume that a woman's libido absolutely pales in comparison to the visceral and mind-consuming lust of their own male sex drive. We do know that testosterone is a huge factor in human sex drive, and us males have ten times as much testosterone as women, so it's fair to say our libido outpaces theirs, right? In a way, yes. The healthy male sex drive always seems to be in the **ON** position, ready to go at a moment's notice. It doesn't take much at all to get fire the engine up. I'll share a personal story that is the perfect illustration of this phenomenon.

One night, soon after a fancy schmancy invitation-only, outdoor farm-to-table seven-course dinner with my wife, my body decided that it needed to hastily evacuate my stomach and all of its expensive hipster-prepared contents. Not sure if it was food poisoning or a virus that I caught from the kids, but I experienced eight straight grueling hours of explosive vomiting and butt-torturing diarrhea. It was not pretty.

As the sun came up the next day, my body was finally done punishing me. I laid in bed a dehydrated and broken shell of a man. It felt like I had been through a war. My wife laid down next to me, naked after a shower. I took one look at her, and my penis took over. I had to have her. She couldn't believe I was capable of conjuring up the energy to get the deed done, but I was. There was no work on her part needed (beyond being naked next to me) to get me into the right headspace necessary to have sex with her right then and there. I saw her body, and I wanted her. She was willing. Sex was had. It didn't matter that I had spent the entire night staring at a toilet filled with the foulest concoction a mind can conjure up. It didn't matter that my muscles were cramping and my lips were dry from dehydration. The only thing that mattered was my penis saying, *"Hey, boss. See that over there? Any particular reason why you're not letting me do my job right now?"*

On the other side of the coin, female libido seems to be much more **responsive** in nature. It may take a certain combination of actions and the right environment to conjure up the emotional and physical cues necessary to get the sex machine turned on, but for most women, the desire IS in there. Many men are under the impression that since their wife often turns down his sexual advances, her sexual desire must be naturally less than his. No, her sexual desire for him at that particular moment was less than his desire for her. Notice I said for HIM. The boiling desire for sex is probably in there, lurking under the surface. The set of circumstances needed to push her sex buttons in the right order and get the machine cranking don't include, *"Seeing my overweight husband in his stained sweat pants burping in the kitchen after eating a PB&J sandwich and drinking his second beer while he fondles my boob"*. It's usually a little more complex than that.

Here's the kicker: **When the buttons are pushed in the right sequence, female sexuality runs laps around male sexuality.** Women are, by nature, much more fluid and *"wild"* (for lack of a better word) with their sexuality. This has been illustrated in the scientific realm by observational studies likes those done at Queens University in Kingston, Ontario. In these studies, they utilized devices connected to subjects' genitalia. These devices specifically measured for blood flow (arousal). When men were asked what they were turned on by, their arousal displayed accordingly. If they said they liked watching naked women having lesbian and hetero sex, they became erect when watching women having sex in porn.

These men did not get aroused when watching gay male porn or when watching animals mating. There was a very definite mind-genital connection at work. The man says what he likes and the penis agrees.

Women, on the other hand, responded positively to a wide array of different visual stimuli. It could be gay porn, straight porn, lesbian porn… sometimes even videos of animals fornicating, and their genitals would swell in apparent physical arousal. BUT, if you asked those same women exactly what they found sexy and arousing, they would respond much like the men. The hetero women said they liked typical heterosexual stimuli, the gay women liked lesbian sex, and no… they certainly do not like to watch animals having sex. Yet, their genitalia seemed to tell a completely different story. It's almost as if their bodies were betraying their minds … or perhaps they were being dishonest out of shame and fear of looking like a sex-hungry nymphomaniac. Maybe a little of both.

Speaking of pornography, it is a fact that the vast majority of porn consumers are male. Men have that sex drive switch in the constant ON AND READY position, after all. When he badly needs relief from a building sexual urge, porn is the quick, easy and free solution. What do men online search for in porn? Usually, it's age-related terms like *"Teen"* or *"Milf"* (youth tends to win over maturity). How about those women that occasionally watch and enjoy porn, what are they searching for? They search for key terms like **lesbians, threesomes, infidelity and group sex. In fact, women are 132% more likely to search for lesbian porn than men. Women also searched for the term** *"gangbang"* **80% more often than men, and** *"threesome"* **75% more often.** Women in their porn searches also show a strong preference for subjects like *rough sex* and *bondage*, way more so than men (a great book about internet porn trends and what they say about us is **A Billion Wicked Thougts**).

CHAPTER 1: WHY DID THIS HAPPEN?

Like I said… the energy is in there.

Want to hear some jaw-dropping true stories about female sexuality? Talk to a male stripper. The male stripper is the center of attention during a very interesting and very heated exhibit of unbridled female sexuality. He's in a room full of women that are there to see man flesh AND (this is the important part, so pay attention) **they all feel free and safe to outwardly demonstrate their arousal**. It's understood that it is A-Okay to scream, grab the stripper, smack his butt, yank at his speedos, laugh, and high-five her friends. Once the usually conservative and sexually boring women in the bachelorette party pick up on the *"Be free and do whatever you want… no judgment here"* vibe in the room, all bets are off. Male strippers will tell you tales of brides-to-be performing oral sex on him in front of her friends, bridesmaids taking off their tops to get the stripper's attention, women jerking off the stripper while friends cheer her on, etc. The frenzy of the moment is so intense, that some women seem to be completely caught off guard by their own body's response to the situation. The boring mom of three can't believe what she just did to some strange man in a room full of screaming women. She was just Suzy Homemaker going to her friend's innocent bachelorette party… and now she's some crazed slut who jerked off the muscular stripper and made out with one of the bridesmaids on a dare. These women are later seen outside crying their eyes out while their friends try to calm them down. *"It's okay, sweetie. We were all stupid. It was a party. Don't worry, he won't find out. Nobody will say anything. We promise."*

The Open Marriage Phenomenon

Female sexuality can be seen as mysterious, dangerous, or maybe even a little silly by some. At the same time, it can be seen as an empowering exhibit of emancipation and self-discovery by others. Generations of female sexual shame and the modern day *"You go girl, do whatever makes you happy for once in your life"* mentality has led to a great deal of confusion and teen-like rebellion by women in intimate relationships today. This rebellion is perfectly illustrated with the dramatic increase in requests for open marriages. **Did you know that women are statistically twice as likely as men to suggest an open marriage?** It shouldn't come as a surprise. Women, by and large, are not excited or turned on within the confines of a standard monogamous marriage. The comfort and familiarity kill their libido, as we now know. Modern day women are starting to become more comfortable letting the sexually frustrated cat out of the bag. *"Ummm... I'm just not turned on anymore. How about I have sex with other men? You can have sex with other women! Win-win!"*

There is no inherent *"problem"* with female sexuality, just as there is no problem with male sexuality. Neither should be shamed into submission. Trying to subdue the natural urge will just push it further underground, but it won't make it go away. In fact, it will just bubble up in a more toxic and unhealthy form. A man may be told to act like a gentleman and to suppress his natural urges and not objectify women... but he will just sneak off to the basement with a laptop and watch porn for hours, and later feel awful about it as he hides his habit from his partner. If you want to be in a relationship with a woman AND have a strong sex life AND keep her faithful, you must understand and appreciate the nuance, subtlety, and fluidity of her sexuality.

The problem (as I see it) comes when the wife recognizes the lack of oomph in her relationship and decides that the best course of action is to take the giant mental and physical leap of suggesting sex with others. This usually happens after already letting her boundaries down and beginning an emotional (or possibly physical) relationship with another man. By asking for permission to be sexual with other men, she is completely skipping the hard, but ultimately rewarding work of making the existing marriage more sexual and fun. There is a myriad of things a couple can do to *"spice things up"* in a marriage, and to jump right to intimate relationships with other people is more than a bit hasty and deconstructive. By suggesting such an arrangement, a woman is advertising her innate desire to seek out more attractive sexual partners and her subsequent lack of respect for her current man.

From a strictly biological point of view, an open marriage for a woman is an understandable and extremely effective solution to a glaring problem: **Her sexual desire for her husband is low and it continues to fade with time.** She wants to feel that intense sexual urge and heightened force of *"new relationship energy"* again. She believes that engaging in an open marriage will reignite the fire and successfully push her buttons again. **She's exactly right. It will.** After all, there is NOTHING that can compare to the energy and lust that is conjured up by the act of engaging in an intimate relationship with a new person. Nothing pushes the sexual engine buttons easier, faster and with more gusto. You, as a human, were programmed to react in this way, and your wife is no different.

This whole *"open marriage"* phenomenon is biological. It's her body saying to her brain, *"My current mate's reproductive use is done. Too many signals are telling me that he is no longer worthy of copulation. Must find a new, more suitable mate."* And then later, *"Oh yes, this new man is perfect! I feel amazing! Must devote all time and energy to new the mate. Drop old mate immediately. Begin the new pair-bonding process."*

The current progressive mindset dictates that open marriages are an understandable and modern (and therefore more enlightened) expression of female sexuality. Women are not the **"property"** of men, after all, and they should feel free to express their sexual urges and have extramarital relations as their body and brain see fit. Society should support them for doing so (if you think I'm exaggerating, do a google search on open marriages). After all, as the arguments go, men have been openly having affairs and girlfriends on the side for generations. It's been an understood and tolerated phenomenon. The wife gets older and more frigid, the high-value man's sexual needs aren't being met, so he goes out and gets some on the side. We saw this tolerance famously illustrated in 1996 with the funeral for former French President François Mitterrand. Both his wife and his mistress attended the funeral, sitting side-by-side, much to the shock of many Americans… and the understanding shrug of many Europeans. *"What's the big deal? Men have affairs. He still supported his wife and children and he still ran the nation of France longer than anyone else in history."*

As sexist as it sounds, I have yet to see a female-driven *"open marriage"* succeed long-term. In every single case that I am personally aware of, the end is the same: **The wife eventually bonds with another man and leaves the husband.** She may explain that she didn't INTEND to *"catch feelings"* for the guy, it just happened. As one reader of my site shared, his wife came to him proclaiming her feelings for one of the men she slept with during their open marriage. The husband quickly pointed out that they now have an open marriage, so what's the big deal? Isn't that, after all, the point of the open marriage? You get to keep your marriage intact and go out and have fun with others, right? She responded by saying that her new partner was NOT in favor of open marriages. He wanted her all for himself, so she had to leave her marriage to be with the new lover. She disconnected from the husband, she bonded with another man, she divorced the husband. That seems to be the standard series of events in the modern-day world of open marriages.

Who Cares?

What does all of this stuff like female sexuality and human behavior, in general, have to do with you, a guy who was dumped by his long-term partner? Well, just about everything. With all of this knowledge in hand, you are able to better understand exactly what happened to you, and more importantly, how to avoid it happening again with a new partner. You see, you may not know it right at this moment, but your brain is going to want you to connect with another woman (or women) and form another intimate relationship pretty damn quickly. You're going to want to date, and you're going to soon become attached all over again. You can't help it, it's in your biology. Due to your history, you are especially prone to the charms of another woman. You have a deep psychological wound that you need to tend to, and nothing *"heals"* that faster than another woman. As they say, *"If you want to get over a woman, get under another one."* It's a funny saying, but it's an incredibly unhealthy path to go down.

The statistics show that you have a better than 50/50 chance of fucking it up, divorcing, and doing this whole horrible recovery process all over again. You need to understand what you're up against. Your life may depend on it.

Chapter 2: Real Love

Up until now, a romantic relationship and finding the coveted gold ring of "Real Love" is probably something that you haven't put a whole lot of time, thought or planning into. You probably believe that it eventually *"just happens"* to most men, much like catching a cold or taking a dump. *"Men date around a little, find the love of their life, get married and have kids. That's just the way it is"* readers will often tell me. They tell me romantic stories about how their grandparents met and are still together so many decades later. Grandpa saw Grandma at the corner store buying candy when they were both twelve years old. He knew right then and there he would marry her, and he eventually did. It's been sunshine, rainbows and lots of grandkids ever since.

Most men don't treat finding new relationship partners like the dramatic life-changing experiences that they truly are. In fact, men will put more time into finding the right car with the right options than they will put into finding the right partner for life. When car hunting, they'll research different models, compare used versus new, look at different financing options, look at the additional cost of the heated seats and rear-facing camera, consider an extended warranty, etc. With a relationship, they simply fall for that cute girl that showed them interest that one time.

"Hey, Sally from accounting is cute and she likes me. Cool. Wonder what she'd be like as a wife..."

Unlike what popular culture tells us, men tend to be hopeless romantics in relationships. Any hint of pragmatism goes out the window when it comes to interacting with the fairer sex. Most men truly feel that Real Love just miraculously falls from the sky. They also feel that women think in the same way.

They couldn't be more wrong.

What is "Real Love"?

Real Love is a choice. Real Love is a sacrifice. Real Love is something that two people have to work hard to achieve and maintain throughout the course of a long-term relationship. Real Love is extremely rare. Chances are you won't experience true Real Love in your lifetime. Most of you won't.

Oh sure, you will experience a crush, overwhelming lust, and nervous butterflies over a girl. We all have that from time to time. The feelings may be reciprocated, and you may end up in a monogamous relationship that will last years. You may have kids, a mortgage, shared assets, etc. The delicate nature of your relationship eventually shows its ugly self when shit hits the fan, or something dramatically changes the dynamic of your marriage. It could be something simple like a job change, promotion, job loss, or the death of a parent. Sometimes that is all it takes to get the divorce train rolling. The boundaries are broken down and a series of psychological events change your spouse's mindset completely. One minute you're thinking about what to make the kids for dinner, and the next minute your wife is crying about how she just doesn't have feelings for you anymore.

It happens.

Sorry if this happened to you, but what you had wasn't Real Love. It was a chapter in your life that resulted in a lot of great memories and a lot of sadness. You're not the first to think he was in a Real Love relationship and you won't be the last. We've all been fooled at one time or another. Such is life.

The timeline of a good Real Love relationship:

• Super strong mutual physical attraction.
• Flirting. Getting to know each other. Sex. Strong sexual compatibility.
• *"Wow, I really like this person a great deal. Both inside and out. I'd like to try a monogamous relationship with them."*
• Years of a strong relationship.
• Genuine love, respect, and appreciation. Strong bond. True partnership.
• Marriage.
• Children.
• Struggle. Bad Times.
• Enduring love and devotion.
• Grandkids. Great grandkids.
• Death.

It's somewhere around the *"Struggle"* part where a lot of relationships are exposed for what they really are. The men I talk to are proud to say that they stuck it out and worked hard during the really tough times of their marriage. Unfortunately, with hindsight being 20/20, the man realizes that the tough times are exactly when things started to go south for their wife. She just wasn't nearly as tough as he thought she was. He later learns that nobody ever taught her how to cope when shit hit the fan. She also never learned the concept of *"boundaries"* while growing up. She was far too pliable with her emotions, bending whichever way the wind blew. Eventually, she was mentally overwhelmed by the inevitable awfulness and boredom that life dishes out to all of us. She attempted to relieve her anxieties in the worst way. She let nature and her compulsions take over.

She may have shopped until the credit cards maxed out. She may have eaten until she gained 100 lbs. She may have texted her ex-boyfriend and sent him nude photos. She may have had an affair with her asshole coworker. All of these things are a form of self-medicating and attempts to drown out what she innately knows: **She doesn't have it in her to maintain a Real Love relationship.** She's just not cut out for it. She doesn't have the right tools in her mental toolbox. She's just a common broken human being.

Contrary to popular belief, Real Love is not for all of us. It's funny how we are quick to say, *"Running a marathon is not for me"* or *"Being a rocket scientist is not for me"* … but I'll be damned if nearly everyone doesn't think they have God-given RIGHT to a long-term Real Love relationship. A combination of peer/family pressure and Hollywood fiction have convinced us that falling for somebody and being together forever and ever is the magic endgame for absolutely everyone. Yes, everyone knows about the awful divorce statistics, but what's the first thing we all say when somebody breaks up? *"You'll find somebody again! Trust me!"* We treat the end goal of finding a Real Love life partner just like going to the bathroom or eating food. It's a given that you need it and will find it.

For most people, Real Love is just too damn hard to maintain. It takes two to tango, as they say. What most don't tell you is that it takes an entire family and social circle to help you keep the relationship machine humming away, as well. Unfortunately, you can't just assume that all of your partner's family and friends will have your relationship's best interests in mind. If your spouse is dangling on the edge of the divorce cliff, more than a few people close to her are waiting to gleefully push her right on over and watch her plummet to her relationship death. In today's society, there is a chorus of people that will cheer on your wife's bad decisions. They will gladly give the worst advice that ends up dramatically ending your marriage, much to the confusion of the betrayed husband. What you don't see is that your wife is a beacon of hope for her bored friends who dream of saying *"fuck it"* and walking away from their own god-awful marriages. They will live vicariously through your wife's bad girl behavior and enjoy every drama-filled moment.

Combine society's current *"no judging, no shame"* attitude, a bevy of women who dream of joining the *"walk away wife"* in her new fantastic life, and the growing world of mobile apps that allow relationship-ending behavior to occur with the swipe of a thumb… and it's a recipe for relationship disaster. The good news is that all of these temptations are an excellent way to weed out the bad relationship candidates. The relationships that are left are as strong as you can get. They can endure just about anything and they recognize the power they have when working together as a team. That's everyone's dream.

The bad news is that this strong relationship dynamic represents a very small portion of the population. Your ex-wife, statistically, was not meant to be in a Real Love relationship. Most of us don't find out until after several kids and many years go by. As you now know, most bad relationship candidates don't show their true self until shit hits the fan.

Remember: Most relationship candidates are, in fact, BAD Real Love relationship candidates.

Every Man Thinks He Can Win the Relationship Lottery

Finding and nurturing a Real Love relationship means that a lot of different things need to happen:

1. Finding somebody you are insanely physically attracted to, and

vice-versa.

2. Discovering that you are sexually compatible.

3. Learning that you are emotionally, intellectually and spiritually compatible.

4. Both of you are tough, have good coping skills, and are willing to work through obstacles that life throws at you, together, as a team.

5. Both of you have a good sense of boundaries and are able to resist temptation and compulsive behavior for the good of the partnership and the family.

Note the use of the term *"BOTH"*. Real Love is not a one-person job. Both people have to work in tandem. Both people have to put in time and effort. All it takes is one person to have a hiccup, and the whole thing is over faster than you can say *"I love you but I'm not in love with you"*. It takes two people to marry, but it only takes one person to divorce. The one strong person is not enough to keep things afloat. Yes, I'm talking to you Mr. Fixer Upper guy. You can't fix and maintain a relationship all by yourself.

If you DO find Real Love and you go to your death bed knowing you found your soul mate… congratulations. You won the love lottery. There is absolutely positively nothing better in life. I wish everyone in the world could experience Real Love. It's a magical and wonderful thing. For the vast majority of you reading this, you're not going to find it. I know that's really tough to hear, but it's the truth. I'm not going to bullshit you. You get enough of that from everyone else in your life.

Staying with the lottery analogy, you're going to keep buying scratch-off tickets with hopes of quitting your job and buying that fancy house with the Ferrari in the garage. Sure, every now and then you may scratch off a $500 winner. It's just enough to keep you coming back for more. In the end, the casino always wins. You would've been better off investing that money in yourself. Instead of spending money and time on rolling the relationship dice, you should've joined a gym, invested in yourself, and helped out your community. In the long run, this usually ends up being a cheaper and far more rewarding course of action. Ironically, this is also the course of action that is more likely to lead to a true Real Love relationship.

You Don't NEED Real Love

You need to remove the *"I need to find Real Love or else I'm a failure in life"* mentality from your head. It is just setting yourself up for a miserable life of chasing the promise of the elusive Real Love paradise. When men have the end goal of Real Love in mind, they tend to put up blinders to all the nagging little and not-so-little bad things about our mate we like to call *"red flags"*. All those warning signs that say, *"Uh oh, this is not going to end well for you, dude, take action now,"* are ignored for the greater good of maintaining course to reach the coveted destination of Real Love. It's like the Titanic trying to make record time across the Atlantic and ignoring all the warnings about icebergs in the water. How'd that turn out for them?

The whole mindset of, *"Must find partner, get a house, have a kid before I am 35"* is the typical (and understandable) mindset of a single woman. By no means should you feel pressured to follow suit. Women have the all-powerful biological clock ticking (their growing need for kids along with lowering fertility as they get older) and the consistent societal pressure to make a family of her own. They see their friends spitting out kids and marrying great Provider men with high social status, and dammit, they deserve the same thing!

REMEMBER: Some women are so desperate for the life they "deserve", they will have no hesitation about lying and manipulating to achieve it.

You, as a man, don't have the same innate biological pressure to settle down. Don't ever forget it. Regardless of what your family or friends may tell you, there's zero reason why you should feel that time is ticking away from you. There's no rush whatsoever. Take your time and do it right. You are a man. The women aren't going anywhere, trust me. You should feel free to live life as you choose with no pressure to commit to one woman just because your social circle thinks you should. There is entirely too much at stake to *"settle"* for that one gal that has more red flags than a Chinese parade. Do relationships the right way, or don't do them at all.

Many broken and mentally ill women have a long line of destroyed men in their wake. Every single one of these poor saps thought that they were in a *"Real Love"* relationship with a fantastic woman who they were damn lucky to have for the rest of their life. They couldn't wait to settle down with her and start a life together. In reality, they were just a pawn in a very sick and manipulative game. **She was never his, it was just his turn.**

The Times They Are a-Changin'

Grandparents with marriages that lasted until the day they died had a very strong sense of partnership. They were in it together. Yes, they had fights. They had disagreements. The bedroom wasn't always the lust-filled playground that they both wanted. Life kicked them in the teeth, and they persevered.

Men often like to tout the good ol' days of their grandparents' generation as the Shangri La of marriage past. Men worked. Women stayed home. Divorce rates were very low. Families stayed intact. Yes, it's true, it was a different time. What we don't see is the unfulfilled mom home with kids but no sense of her true self. We don't see the depressed woman whose emotional and physical needs were routinely ignored. We don't see the woman who has absolutely zero options in life other than, ***"Suck it up, make dinner, clean the house and raise the kids into normal productive humans".*** If she were to give up on the marriage and divorce her husband, she would be ostracized by her community. She would be left with nothing. She would be broke with no family and no friends. Is it any wonder the family unit stayed together?

Wives now have many more options in life. They have a much higher sense of financial and overall personal self-worth. Women currently make up the majority of college graduates and regularly earn positions high up the corporate ladder. It is not uncommon for the woman to bring home the bacon while the husband stays home tending to the house and kids. Regardless of what proponents of the *"wage gap"* theory may state, when all things are equal (time at work, experience, education, etc.) … women are neck and neck with men in the workplace, and in many ways surpassing them.

For those women who don't earn a good amount more than their spouse, the family courts have made it possible for a woman to leave her marriage, retain majority custody of the kids and earn a steady paycheck of child support, alimony and half the marital assets. **The government, in no uncertain terms, is telling many women that divorce is not only a perfectly acceptable option, but also a potentially lucrative one.**

Did you know **that approximately 70% of all divorces are initiated by women**? Did you know that in couples where the wife has a college degree, 80% of the divorces are initiated by the woman? Modern day women, it would seem, are just not happy and fulfilled within the framework of traditional marriage. The more financial options they have, the less inclined they are to stick around and do the hard work necessary to keep the marriage afloat.

Take their propensity for negative thought (a.k.a. *"neuroticism"* - one of the **five higher-order personality traits**), a persistent *"Is this really the best I can do?"* mentality, a society that tears down all obstacles in way of her fulfillment, AND add potential financial benefit to leaving… and it's no wonder divorce is so damn common today.

These are some huge obstacles in the way of attaining Real Love.

The Great Irony of Love

Love is a lot like the money game. When you have what you need already, more and more real opportunities just seem to come your way. When you are flush with cash after a big business deal, other genuine money-making opportunities always seem to pop up. When you have a lot of self-respect, self-love and a good head on your shoulders, the decent women seem to come out of hiding (you are actually just better at ignoring the broken ones) and you have more opportunity for a genuine relationship with a really good person. This is the great irony of love: Don't need love? Then you get way more opportunities for it. NEED love? You're in for real trouble.

Fact: Broken women are good at finding broken men.

They can sniff out a broken man like a bloodhound looking for a murder suspect on the run. They will find you. They will manipulate you. They will completely fool you. Don't underestimate their chameleon-like abilities for one second.

Here is the common relationship timeline I hear again and again from my readers:

• A very nice, sweet guy (most likely raised only by mom or without a strong father figure) with relatively little sex/dating experience meets a woman that takes his breath away. ***"It's as if time stopped and an angel came from heaven."***

• She is overly sweet, kind and sexual.

• She has a great deal more sexual experience than he has.

• He falls for her immediately and changes everything in his life for her. Friends, hobbies, interests and career all come second to the new girl.

• Red flags galore. They are ignored for the greater good of continuing the relationship.

• They marry and have kids.

• Red flags start to surface more and more. Ignored again.

• She becomes more jealous and abusive.

• She is either formally diagnosed or is suspected of having Borderline Personality Disorder.

• He is put through the worst kind of relationship hell imaginable.

• She cheats. They divorce. The abuse continues.

All of the above was born out of the man's NEED for

the elusive Real Love. He put a product out there on the market (himself), he marketed it by showing off its attributes (his Provider traits and lack of self-esteem), and the buyers came calling (crazy women). It's that simple.

Chapter 3: Succeeding in Relationships

Thinking about dating again? Ready to get back on the saddle? You're probably not ready. Seriously. I've talked to so many guys who make the mistake of jumping into the dating world way too soon after their separation/divorce from their wife. They will tell me how it's "been a long time" since they have had sex (dead bedroom marriages are common before discovering infidelity and the subsequent divorce) and they just want to get their natural male sexual urges out of their system.

Maybe they just want that close intimate connection with a woman again. Maybe they long for a real-life companion. What they later discover is that they are trying to use women as a psychological bandaid to cover up the massive gaping wound left by their ex. They feel incomplete. They are conditioned to have a woman by their side when going through life, and right now it honestly feels like they lost a limb. They miss sharing life and their day-to-day routine with a woman. They miss the little inside jokes. They miss the partnership. These are the men that fall in love VERY quickly with the first girl that makes goo goo eyes at them, more often than not with disastrous results.

If you're reading this book, you are most likely not ready to date. You are still in too much pain and too broken to bring another human into your life. It's not fair to you, to your family or to the person you are dating. The manic high you will experience when the first woman shows interest in you will be drowned out by the intense low you will feel when it all comes crashing down and ends horribly. You will take one step forward and nineteen steps back. You'll end up worse off than you are now.

You ain't ready, amigo. Trust me.

But, if you're like the vast majority of the men I help, you won't listen to my advice. You'll put up an online dating account or go hang out at the singles bar. Probably both. You'll either become disgusted and depressed about the shallowness of the dating landscape (and the lack of attention you will receive), or you'll become elated at how easy you can get attention and affection from decent looking, seemingly normal women. Regardless of the outcome, if you're like 100% of the men I help, you'll later wish you had waited a while longer before you jumped into the awfulness of the dating pool. All of these men come back to me with their tail between their legs. *"Well, that was stupid."* Hey, people have to learn the hard way. It's human nature. I understand completely. I was one of them.

If you plan on entering the dating world, you need to be aware of just how NOT "normal" and wholesome of an experience it is. You need to be aware that it is, in fact, a giant stupid game. You need to know the rules, the customs and the culture of the stupid game before you jump into it head-first. If you go in blind, you'll just end up as another piece of roadkill on the dating highway.

Do yourself a favor and throw away all your past conceptions of what dating is. Whatever you do, don't bring into this world your notions of "comfort" and "being in a relationship" that you cultivated while you were married. That world in your mind has nothing to do with this new world you're about to dive into. This is dating. If you had prior experience with dating (years ago before you were married), you can throw out all that experience as well. Dating is nowhere near the same as it used to be. Not even close. To be honest, you were probably wrong about the dating game back then, too. That might be part of what got you into this mess in the first place.

The Ugly Truth of the Modern-Day Mating Game

The human mating game begins with and is primarily based upon basic animalistic attraction. It's visual. We want what looks good to us. The whole process starts with *"Whoa. Who is THAT*

over there?" In today's online dating landscape, this "shallow" visual mindset is more obvious than ever. Don't think for one second that the "good" women in online dating see right past your looks and dig deeper into your profile to discover your "true" good qualities. Sorry, no. It's never been that way and never will be that way. **Your looks get you in the door. Your personality keeps you there.**

There's a somewhat disturbing but oh-so-true phenomenon that society has known for generations now, but we haven't really quantified to any certain degree. We all know this to be true, but we never could put a real number on it. Now, thanks to the anonymous data-driven nature of the internet, we have the numbers to illustrate the ugly truth:

Women find 80% of the men on the dating market to be unattractive.

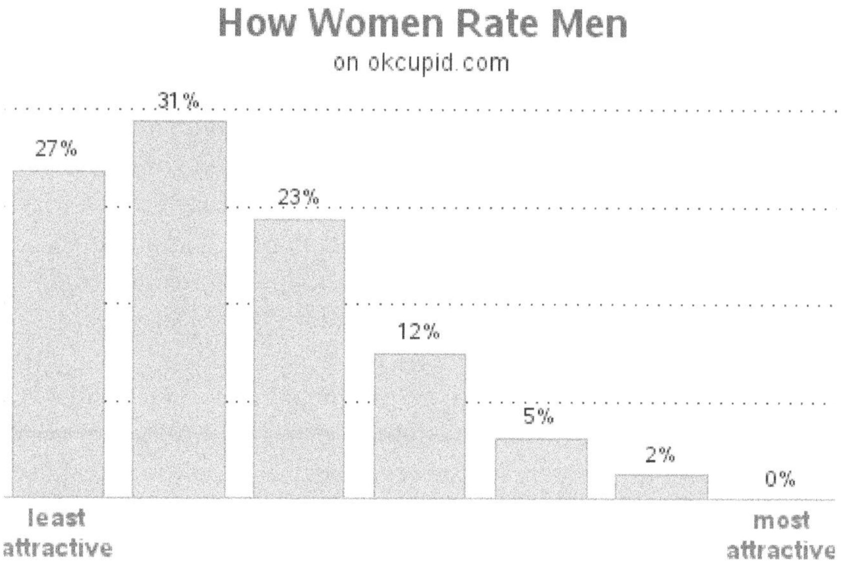

Men, on the other hand, tend to have a more "fair" distribution of who is attractive, average and unattractive.

How Men Rate Women
on okcupid.com

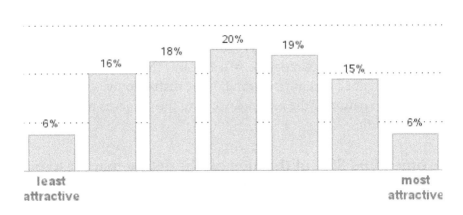

Conclusion: Women are very picky. Men… not so much. Again, we all knew this already. A man will bang almost anything that gives him the time of day, and women will try to hold out for the best possible man they can get. Men have to put on a show of qualifying himself to earn the reward of a woman's time. The women in question don't have to be a super-attractive top-tier woman, either. They just need to be available. We all know super high-value men that routinely sleep with objectively average and below average women. The super stud had needs, the so-so gal from the bar was available, they had sex.

To summarize: Women on the complete spectrum of the attraction scale get sexual access to the top-tier men. Whether she's a perfect 10 or the homely housekeeper, she has a legitimate chance at a night of fun. Women have a buffet of mate choices. They can be picky. Men, on the other hand, will take what they can get. In comparison, the sexual menu is limited for men. Yes, the mating game is, and always has been, a woman's market.

Even with the data in our face, people will disagree: *"Yes, but if that were true, then why are all these women marrying men left and right? If they only like 20% of the guys at a visceral attraction level, then there aren't enough guys to go around and very few women would be in relationships and eventually marry."*

The answer is simple: **Women often settle.** In the interest of fulfilling their desire to have babies and attain financial and emotional security, women will "settle" for a man that is in the 80% group. She will weigh the pros and cons and convince herself that he is "good enough". Sure, she longs for the 20% guy with the great looks, personality, and charisma that makes her underwear fly off… but that's obviously super rare in a guy and not realistic. If she wants to start up that family life she always dreamed about, she better set aside her dreams of the knight in shining armor and give those good-but-not-perfect guys a chance. Unfortunately, this common theme of "settling" or "giving up" on finding Mr. Perfect keeps some women operating with a consistent undercurrent of resentment. *"Nothing I do is ever good enough for her"* men in these relationships will say. It's true. The man had two strikes against him before he even stepped up to the plate. He feels like he has to consistently qualify himself and prove his worth, because he does.

Don't Make Dating and Marriage Your Life's Mission

Dating should only be approached as a fun diversion in life. It should be ancillary to your mission, your friends, your self-care and your family. Dating should never be approached with the end game of marriage and attaining Real Love in mind. You just want to meet nice, fun and attractive women to spend time with. That's it. You want to go into this with the mindset of a **Mentally Healthy Non-Needy Man (MHNNM)**.

The MHNNM realizes that most women he dates will not be long-term relationship material. They won't even come close. They will be varying degrees of broken women, mentally ill women, and really good women who unfortunately were never given the tools to learn how to be successful in a long-term relationship. A chosen few MAY be up for the job as your life partner, but they will be the rare exception to the rule.

The MHNNM may eventually decide to try out a monogamous relationship with a seemingly good woman. If he does so, he makes sure to keep his eyes and ears open for signs that her behavior would be detrimental to his wellbeing. If real red flags are detected, he hits the eject button and bails out of the relationship with no hesitation and no animosity. *"I like you a lot. I appreciate your time, but this isn't going to work out for me. I wish you nothing but the best."*

Unfortunately, what many experienced MHNNM men will tell you is that they hit that eject button over and over and over again… and it grows tiresome. Eventually, they grow cynical and lose faith in the whole monogamous process. They tell their dates right up front, *"Just so you know, I'm not interested in a serious long-term relationship."* It's honest, mature and refreshing, but also a huge disappointment to a large number of women looking to settle down with a great guy they caught in an ocean of awful men. *"All men care about is sex with no commitment"*, they will say.

It's not that the men don't want to commit, or that they have an unnatural *"fear of commitment"* (a common shaming tactic by women in the MHNNM's social circle). The vast majority of men that I talk to have a very real desire to be in a comfortable, long-term relationship with the woman of their dreams. Unfortunately, that woman remains in his dreams. She's rarely found out in the real world. It's not a matter of being "unrealistic" or having

74

"ridiculously high standards", as many people will tell the bachelor (a projection of the common female mindset), but it's instead a matter of recognizing that mental illness, poor life choices, terrible childhoods, laziness, several illegitimate children, and lack of ambition are all signs of a person that is not suitable for the extremely important and difficult job of "life partner". They could be a great friend, they may be great for the occasional date, but they're not somebody you say "I do" to. That's just asking for a shit ton of trouble, as many of us later learn years down the line.

It's the poor quality of the available female partner candidates that keeps the MHNNM in perpetual bachelorhood. The MHNNM recognizes the life-ruining power that the wrong woman can have, so he treads very carefully. He's not desperate. He's not one of the 80% that is DYING for female attention and will gladly hand over his time and resources to them. The MHNNM never settles. He never brushes red flags under the rug and hopes they go away. This is a perfectly healthy mindset, and not one worthy of any shame or guilt.

Never Be Ashamed to be the MHNNM

A lot of men are conditioned to feel guilty about just "having fun" and dating without hastily committing long-term to one woman. After all, what do we mean when we say we are just interested in *"having fun"*? We mean having sex and going out on dates. It means doing all the fun stuff without throwing the proverbial monkey wrench into the machine and watching it explode, just so that you can check off *"in committed relationship"* from your to-do list. It means maintaining sanity, having fun and doing what we can to fulfill our emotional and physical needs and still maintain our life missions and our dignity.

Contrary to popular belief, most men do not want to feel like some kind of sexual predator douchebag that is simply interested in sex with a buffet of strange women. The MHNNM doesn't want to be seen as the guy who has zero regards for women's emotions. They just want to be honest, drama-free and, yes, have their needs met... but they still strive to be a decent human being with a good heart. Society will tell the MHNNM again and again that it's an impossible task.

Trying to maintain this good-hearted single MHNNM persona is really difficult for most guys. It certainly doesn't help that all of the women (and even some men) in a man's life are brow-beating him and attempting to shame him into a more "stable" and comfortable life with one woman. *"When are you going to settle down and meet a nice girl?"* mom will say at Christmas dinner. *"You know, a real man wouldn't date a bunch of girls... he would commit to one. Like that Mary gal you were dating last year. She was a doll,"* Aunt Teresa will say while you're waiting in line for birthday cake. Every MHNNM hears it again and again. Why are all people in his life doing this? What are they REALLY trying to tell him? Why is it that being a single man and having fun is such a turnoff to so many people in his social circle?

What they are all really telling you is that they would much prefer you be seen in the comfortable, "safer", more "respectful", and more "productive" role as the Provider. They don't want to see you as a sexual being. They don't want to think of their son/nephew/cousin/brother as the "Lover" who jumps from woman to woman and doesn't truly contribute to society overall (based on their own preconceptions of personal value and what "contribution" entails).

Lover vs. Provider

In the mating game, men can be categorized in one of two ways: He is either the Lover, or he is the Provider. It's not a difficult concept to wrap your mind around. We all know Lovers and Providers in our own life. Maybe we called them Jocks and Dorks in high school. Popular Guys and Nerds. Alpha Males and

Beta Males. Bad Boys and Nice Guys. Whatever you call it, we all innately know what it means. It's a phenomenon as old as time.

The Lover is the fun guy. He's the guy that a girl may date and have lots of crazy sex with, but she probably wouldn't ever bring him home to meet mom and dad. She may show him off to friends, follow him on social media, have long sexting sessions with him, be very sexually open and experimental with him, and skip work or class just to see him… but the idea of marriage and long-term commitment may not even be on the radar with the Lover. A lot of the time, the Lover is actually a bit of a loser. He could live on a mattress on the floor of his parents' basement, drive a shitty car, and be "in between jobs" … but there is something about the guy that drives the women crazy. It could be his looks. His charisma. His charm. His abundance of confidence. Whatever the indescribable IT is, he's got it in spades. He's a natural.

The Provider, on the other hand, is the safe bet. He's the stable guy. He's the one that will probably make a great dad and always be there for his future wife. If you're a woman, you definitely want to bring this guy home to mom and dad. *"See? I know how to pick a good guy! Isn't he the ideal husband you always had in mind for me?!"* The Provider looks absolutely perfect on paper. He checks all the boxes. He's good looking enough. He's super nice. He wants to start a family. He has a career. So, what's the problem? The problem is that the Provider is just not a sexy man. At all. He doesn't have that indescribable "it" factor. There's no oomph there. There's no, *"I would drive four hours in a blizzard just to spend the night with him"* there. Nature is not screaming, *"BREED WITH THIS HUNK OF A MAN. MAKE BABY. NOW. BEFORE HE GETS AWAY."* Instead, nature is whispering to the woman, *"He'll probably do a great job of taking care of you and your children."* See the difference? In evolutionary terms, it's not unheard of for the Lover to make the babies and for the Provider to take care of them. Modern scientific advances in cheap DNA

77

testing like 23andMe.com have brought this sad fact to light. Endless Tinder profiles with pregnant 20-something girls looking for a "real man" to settle down with and "no more games" shows this to still be the case. The Lover had his fun, now she needs a Provider to clean up the mess.

The Provider is the guy who frequently complains about his awful married sex life. He's the guy who says that his wife switched off the sex supply and got fat as soon as she said "I do", pulling the marital "bait and switch" routine on him. The Provider longs for passion and lustfulness from his wife. The lack of intimacy and validation kills him inside. He truly loves his wife with all of his heart. He probably has an unhealthy worship of her. He can't fathom cheating on his wife or divorcing her, so he attempts to remedy the situation by trying to appeal to his wife's rational side. He will often have sit-down conversations with her and point out that his physical needs aren't being met. *"I love you, but it's like you don't even LIKE me anymore"* he may say. The "Big Talk" usually just makes things exponentially worse. He is bringing to light the uncomfortable truth that every woman in his wife's position doesn't want to verbalize, much less hear from her own Provider husband: **She is just not turned on by him. She settled for him. That's just how it is.**

The Provider's frigid wife also has very real human sexual needs. They are also not being met. She's miserable. She's constantly reminded of just how much she had to "settle" to be in this marriage, yet she will rarely admit her frustrations out of fear of losing her Provider. Her sexual atomic bomb will remain undercover and dormant until the day her psychological boundaries are down, and the sexual engine is fired up again. This is normally done with a new Lover.

"I'm Not Like That Anymore"

Here is a common scenario (thanks to the internet) that

further illustrates the difference between Lovers and Providers:

A man in a stable but boring marriage discovers the surprisingly kinky and promiscuous past of what he thought all along was a sexually dull and inexperienced wife. It may be that he found an old USB thumb drive tucked away in a closet and on it was a video of his wife having a threesome with a man and another woman. Maybe he found a series of sexually graphic photos of his wife from several years ago posted on the internet for all to see. Maybe he found a diary or blog with all the sordid details of boyfriends past and their amazing sexual escapades. In these sexual mementos from years gone by, she is seen as being open, free and fun, doing sexual things she says she said she would never ever do with her husband because they are "gross", "silly" or *only for the fake porn people because nobody in real life does stuff like that*".

Sometimes the wife's secret sexual past is revealed by an ex-college boyfriend or sorority sister that the husband meets at a college reunion or at a company Christmas party. After a few drinks, these old friends gladly spill the beans about how his wife was "the biggest slut" back in the day. As the booze flows throughout the night, the stories get more and more graphic. Others are called over to share their own versions of the wife's sexy past. *"Hey, Karen! Remember when Sally fucked that one pizza guy on a dare while you watched and cheered her on?!"* The unsuspecting husband is left feeling like he was hit by a truck. *"MY wife did all THAT?! Seriously?! No way. This has to be some kind of sick joke."*

The end result of these discoveries: The Provider quickly realizes what his role is and always has been in his wife's life… and he feels completely fooled and humiliated. He is both boiling with anger and incredibly sad at the same time. He always hoped that HE was the guy that would have the power to bring out his wife's animalistic sexual side, not some LOSER from her past. He feels like he has been playing the part of the chump this whole time.

He gets the privilege of devoting all of his time, energy, love and resources to the spouse ... and gets relatively little genuine physical intimacy and sexual validation in return. Douchebag McLoserface from college got to have multiple threesomes with her and she SURE seemed to like oral sex back then (along with everything else on the sexual menu).

Once he gets up the nerve to approach his wife with the newfound evidence of her past, she will do her best to put him at ease. She was just in a young "phase" of her life back then, she will explain. She may say that she felt "pressured" to do those things in college because she was young, immature, and thought she would lose her asshole of a boyfriend if she didn't do the threesome, give him oral sex, or pose for the all those photos that were posted on the internet. The husband listens, but he can't drop it. He keeps drilling away with more questions. *"Ok, then what about the pizza guy that Deb told me all about? Did you feel pressure to fuck him, too?! How about the guy you banged while on the trip to France your Freshman year? Or the guy in Spain who wore the matador cape while he banged you at the pool party??"* As his questions and accusations keep coming, his wife's anger starts to build. What does it matter what she did back then? This is NOW, and she loves HIM, not all those losers from her past. She has matured since then. That was YEARS ago. She's a completely different person now. She's a mom and his devoted wife. She chose HIM. He should appreciate and respect that. She shouldn't be judged by some experimental young phase in her life.

With every explanation she gives, the wife just digs herself deeper and deeper into a hole that she won't be able to climb out of. She did the most personal and physically vulnerable acts with people that were "losers" in comparison to her loving husband (in her own words). She didn't form close, intimate bonds with them as she did with her husband. She didn't have children with them. Those men weren't there for her when she had her breast cancer scare, or when she gained 60 lbs with her pregnancy. This makes her husband, in his own mind, less than a loser. He doesn't possess the qualities needed to elicit the same sexual response from the wife he loves more than anyone on Earth. He's completely crushed, and the wife just doesn't seem to get it.

Her lack of empathy towards her husband is completely baffling to him. He's probably never felt a deeper sense of betrayal than in this moment, and his wife's only solution is to further blame him for even questioning her sexual past and current relationship motives. Yet, everything she says just points to the same conclusion: **The other guy(s), along with the free and fun atmosphere of her youth, elicited a level of consistent and heightened sexual energy that marriage and dear boring husband cannot spark for even a few seconds.** She was free, wild, happy and animalistic with THEM… and an asexual boring mom with HIM. He's had to endure years of *"I just feel fat and gross and don't want to do anything"* and *"Can you just give it a rest for one night?"* Those guys from her past just had to show up with some beer and a pizza and she was the instant star in a real-life porn movie.

He is the Provider. Those other men were her Lovers. Age and maturity have nothing to do with it, as many guys like him learn after discovering their wife in a torrid love affair with a douchebag just like the ones she "outgrew" from her fun and free past.

The Elusive Lover+Provider Man

The ideal guy for a woman is one that has both Lover and Provider qualities. He's the charming, ambitious and good-looking guy with the heart of gold. He's the fun, friendly but slightly dangerous guy that other women fantasize about. Women don't look at him and say, *"I wish I could fool him into marrying and providing for me"*. Instead, they say, *"I wish he would PICK ME!"* See the difference? The ideal man is a prize that has his pick of the litter. Think of the TV show "The Bachelor". Women don't settle for The Bachelor (the uber-successful and super handsome young guy with perfect hair). They win him. In fact, oddly enough, they don't mind sharing him, as we learn when watching the Bachelor make out and eventually sleep with girl after girl, only to have them all cry when he doesn't hand them the coveted rose that keeps them on the show. If they get to have their own alone time with Prince Charming and possibly win him in the end, then they can turn a blind eye to all the other "dates" he has with the other pretty contestants. Like the elusive beautiful Unicorn of a woman who has a good heart, solid boundaries, and coping skills that serve her well in a long-term relationship, the good all-around Lover+Provider guy is VERY rare and in VERY high demand. A prime relationship candidate like that is usually snagged early on by a high-value Unicorn. Unfortunately for most 30+ year-old post-divorce women in the dating game (the majority of single women you will encounter), they quickly realize that finding the good all-around L+P guy is damn near impossible. That leaves women with two options: Lover OR Provider. They just can't seem to find both wrapped together in one man.

Single women will likely dabble on both sides of the Lover/Provider fence during their dating career. If they're still in their fertile 20's, they may very likely date solely on the Lover side. Life for the young woman is primarily about FUN and self-discovery, after all. Like most young people, they fall into the stupid "forever young" mentality and put partying and making money ahead of the boring stuff like finding a life partner and making babies. Because of this mindset, they will listen only to their young libido, and that libido is telling them to go for the Lovers that make them swoon, not the Providers you bring home to mom.

But, as we all know, life has a way of sneaking up on you pretty damn fast. The next thing you know, you're a woman celebrating your 30th birthday. Everything begins to change. Your body is not the same. Who is this person in the mirror? Why does my back hurt? Why are my arms suddenly flabby? To make matters worse, it seems like all your friends are married and having babies. Your parents are constantly pressuring you to settle down, which is the last thing you need to hear. *"Yeah, like it's such an easy task for a 30-year-old woman to find a perfect life partner! You just go to the husband store and pick one out, right?!"*

Then, in what feels like just a few short years later, you're suddenly 40. You're left wondering what in the hell just happened. This isn't funny anymore. This is downright depressing. This is the sad reality for many single women in the modern dating game.

The Career Gal

More than a few women in my social circle find themselves with great careers but no prospects for a long-term "Real Love" relationship, let alone concrete plans for having children they so desperately NEED to have. With the biological clock screaming at them, these women finally wake up and start dating with the goal of finding a long-term partner. They make the mistake of overestimating the quality of the available male dating pool (L+P men are very rare) AND they way overestimate their own value as a long-term partner. When somebody asks them what their own positive qualities are, they start listing their Ph.D, their awesome career, their apartment in the city and the vacation condo in Florida. They're ironically taking a page from the Provider book of dating tips, and they think it will result in the perfect Lover+Provider partner they so assuredly "deserve".

Nope. Not gonna happen.

As I said before, most of the Lover+Provider guys are off the market. They may have already settled into a stable relationship back in their twenties, or they have been around the block more than a few times and know the rules of the game. In the mind of the L+P man, there's zero incentive to partner with the typical single 30+ year-old gal who finally needs to "settle down" and make a family. In the shallow and unfair world of the dating game, the aging but single L+P guy can actually gain access to the top tier of the female attractiveness pyramid. He is still able to snag the twenty-something attractive women who are just starting out in their relationship journey. In other words, he has his pick of the litter... and Sally the 38-year-old Vice President of Sales for Acme Corporation making $200k per year is not even in the running. Instead, he dates the cute and bubbly barista who just recently graduated from college and still lives with her parents. It's not because the older woman's career is intimidating. Her career is a complete non-factor.

It's not "fair". It sucks for the good, honest and decent women who have worked hard and have a lot to offer in a relationship with a good man. But this is dating. This is the mating game. It's never been fair. It can be unbelievably cruel... as you will probably soon find out for yourself.

No Lover+Provider Guys Available? Time for Plan B.

"Where have all the good men gone?!" women will scream. Translation: *"Where are the good Lover+Provider guys that I feel like a genuinely deserve?"* If they can't find the very rare Lover+Provider guy, they will move on to the next best thing: **The Super Provider.** This change in direction widens their dating pool significantly. Instead of putting things like attractiveness, personality and sexual compatibility at the front of the "must have" list, you will see items like job, money, social status, health and agreeableness at the forefront. Simply put, she's looking for a financially dominant but emotionally submissive man. This man,

much like an actor in a movie, is filling a role in her life plan. She's the director of this movie, and she needs an actor with specific qualifications and skills… and at the same time, they must also be good at taking direction. She has had this life plan in place for many years, and just because she's now past her prime and short on husband candidates doesn't mean it won't happen. Oh, it will happen, even if that means doing things like setting aside her sexual needs or giving up completely on the dream of landing the one Lover+Provider guy. If push comes to shove, she can get her Lover needs met elsewhere.

Unlike what a lot of men may want to believe, most of these "desperate" women don't end up with twelve cats and a drinking problem. Most end up married. Make no mistake, there is a bevy of male Super Providers more than ready and willing to scoop up a desperate single woman and play the part of her hero.

A Lot of Men Are ONLY Comfortable in the Provider Role

A typical recently-divorced man will create an online dating profile (or two, or three) and immediately highlight their Provider qualities. This is the natural game plan that they have fallen back on for years. If he's ever been asked what makes him a good husband, he instantly points out his Provider traits. He's great with kids. He coaches all of their teams. He has a stable job with a good income. He can keep a house clean and well-maintained. He's the kind of guy who loves helping people out when they need it. He's your quintessential "nice guy", in other words.

What is he NOT saying with all of this nice guy Provider behavior? *"I'm a sexual guy who likes to have fun and I know my worth."* This, on the other hand, is precisely what the Lover does. The Lover, in action and words, conveys the theme of, *"I'm awesome. Take it or leave it. I really don't give a shit what you think.*" The Provider, on the other hand, is just like those South American birds you see on the nature shows, doing his little dance while fluffing his feathers and showing off the nest he made while the female stands on her perch feigning interest. *"Pick me! Pick me! Please!"* This is exactly what most men do when dating today. They're telling the women of the world that they KNOW they're not worth much on their own without all their resources. They have nothing other than their Provider qualities to showcase to would-be girlfriends. They might as well provide their credit card number, bank statement and sperm count instead of a headshot on their dating profile.

So, what if you really DO want to play the part of Provider and you don't feel at all comfortable in the Lover role? Well, then I strongly suggest you find a good hobby, get a dog and leave dating alone until you grow into a more well-rounded man. Why? Because you WILL be chewed up and tossed aside like the resource machine that you are. You WILL have your heart crushed and your wallet drained. You WILL be worse off than you were before. It may take years, but it will happen. That's just the way it is in the modern-day relationship game. Nice guys do, in fact, finish last.

What's In Store for the Provider in a Relationship

Once the single woman achieves her goal of landing the Provider, it won't take much time before resentment grows and her feelings of being spiritually, emotionally and sexually unfulfilled grow as well. This is when wives close the sexual gates (*"Not tonight, I have a headache"*), seem to be perpetually angry (nothing you do is ever good enough for her), spend way too much money, and gain fifty pounds. They're not happy. They're miserable. They're trying to fill a void. They're coping (poorly). Nothing about this marriage turned out how they thought it would. The movie is not going according to plan, and the director is pissed off. That's when it's time to fire some actors. As you probably know, it only takes one person in the relationship to step away and call it quits. It's not put up to a democratic vote.

Remember, women file 70 - 80% of all divorces. They have no hesitation to hit the eject button. The Provider is always the one left wondering what in the hell just happened. He did everything right! He played by the imaginary book of rules that he was taught his whole life, and in the end, it bit him on the ass.

If it helps push the point even further, think of what your marriage would be like if you settled for a really nice, kind-hearted woman that was 400 lbs and looked like John Madden. She may be a great conversationalist, may be an awesome friend, and she may be the best mom on the planet… but you would always have this awful ugly cloud hanging over your head. You married an objectively hideous beast of a human being. She doesn't turn you on in the slightest. In fact, she repulses you. You yourself aren't bad looking and other WAY more attractive women flirt with you and they even sometimes bluntly ask you, *"What on EARTH are you doing with HER?!"*

Sound like a marriage made in heaven? Sound like something that has long-term potential? Of course not. Eventually, the man will go crazy or start having emotional and physical affairs with other women… all because something crucial (physical attraction) is missing from his relationship. This is precisely how the woman married to a Provider feels. There's something crucial missing, and she will eventually grow resentful of the mismatch and find ways to fill the void.

Be More Like a Woman

So, what's the point of all this talking about women and their relationship motivations? Isn't this a book geared towards men? Well, yes, but it's good to know what you're up against. It's also good to learn a thing or two from women and use it in your own arsenal of dating weaponry. Women have the dating thing down to a science, and it's time men do the same.

I've said it again and again… Men are the romantics in relationships. They truly believe that women will love them solely for their personality, kindness, and good-heartedness. Many men refuse to believe that while their wife DOES truly love them, it absolutely is a CONDITIONAL love (as it should be). She's not your mother, after all. She's your romantic partner. There ARE conditions that can lead to the shut-down of the relationship. Unfortunately, the conditions are sometimes WAY simpler than what many men want to acknowledge. We always assume since we don't emotionally/physically abuse or neglect our spouse in any way that everything is good to go. We think our sweet nature keeps the evil temptations away from our relationships. Not even close.

Wives have a checklist for actors in the husband/father role in her life movie. If one or more of her needs on the checklist aren't routinely being met, her "must procure new mate" behavior switch is flipped, and the "detaching from my husband" machine starts cranking away. She'll be looking for a new actor to fill the role in no time at all. Many men will throw their hands up in disgust and see this as an example of typical female fickleness ruining a perfectly good lifelong relationship. Yes, it's true that in many ways women are more emotion-driven and have certain behavioral tendencies and personality traits (like higher rates of neuroticism), but when it comes to choosing a mate to partner with for life, they can be surprisingly cold and stoic in their approach. Many men who have lost their job or became physically injured quickly discovered just how disloyal and cruel their wife can be under the right circumstances.

I always tell men that they must TRY to exercise their rational brain muscle and be more like women in relationships, specifically when it comes to choosing and maintaining a relationship with another person. We must be steadfast and strong and keep our eyes and ears open for the bad things that can not only bring down the relationship but also ruin our lives completely. We must develop our own list of "must haves" for a partner and STICK TO IT no matter what. We must be as cold and calculating as the fairer sex has no fear of being.

While she may say, *"Oh, you lost your job? I don't think this is going to work out"*, you are also free to say, *"Oh, you have been diagnosed with depression and borderline personality disorder... I don't think this will work for me"* or *"I see that you are unemployed and have two kids. No thanks! Not interested!"* In other words, stop putting the women on a pedestal and realize that they are flawed human beings and most likely not a good match for you. Don't be afraid to put your needs first. Be the bad guy. Be the asshole. Look past her intoxicating feminine charms and see her for what she may be: A flawed human being who can flush you and everything you love down the toilet.

I know... easier said than done. It's so very tough to not get washed away by the hormones and feel-good chemicals that overwhelm our brains in the presence of a woman, especially one that seems to be so physically and emotionally compatible with you. As they say, when you have the rose-colored glasses on, all the red flags just look like flags. You won't be the first man fooled by the sweet siren song of a beautiful woman, and you certainly won't be the last. It's just part of the game. You need to learn the rules of this game or you WILL get ruined.

Neediness

If there is one thing you need to eliminate TODAY from your single dating persona, it is your neediness. Yes, you are probably a needy person. We all are to some degree. If you're a recently cheated-on divorced guy who just wants to be loved... your neediness is probably through the roof and immediately apparent to everyone in your social circle. For your platonic friends and potential romantic partners, it is absolutely a HUGE turnoff.

89

Nothing is more of a repellant than male behavior that says, *"I NEED you, your attention, your love, and your affection"*. There's a whole collection of awful behavior that comes with neediness, and people just naturally shy away from it. Unless, of course, the other person is mentally ill or severely broken themselves, then they FEED upon your neediness like a pit-bull on a steak. This is precisely why super nice guys always seem to attract the biggest psychos.

Thanks to the growing normalcy of broken families and abusive childhoods, you can't swing a dead cat without hitting a woman with abandonment issues or full-blown Borderline Personality Disorder. These women NEED to be NEEDED and they latch on to broken men like an alien face-hugger. When you put forward your Provider qualities in hopes of snagging a mate, you are inherently advertising your neediness. You are putting up a giant neon sign that says, *"Broken? Nobody else will touch you with a ten-foot pole? Tired of jumping from man to man? Look no further! I'm your knight in shining armor! I will look right past all your glaring faults! Plus... I have stuff I will gladly give you! Money! Time! Lots of love and affection! What are you waiting for?! Please, just give me a chance."* Mentally ill women that are completely ignored by the MHNNM will flock to you, and then discard you like a used napkin.

Social Anxiety

A good number of men that are fresh out of divorce try to throw themselves out there in the dating world, and quickly report back just how much of a stressful and negative emotional experience it was. To quote a reader from my Facebook group:

"Was with the ex for 20 years, since we were 16, and she was my only sexual partner. I'm hoping to start to experience some good stuff going forward. Just feel so socially awkward and anxious

around people. Was at my first ever singles night last week and hated it. Hardly spoke to anyone and convinced myself I'd be alone forever."

What is happening for guys like this reader is one of two things:

1. **They realize that they've always been anxious around other people.** They've been effectively hiding in the cocoon of their marriage all these years, using their wife as a psychological crutch and outlet for their emotions and vulnerabilities that they don't feel comfortable sharing with the rest of the world. They never really put themselves out there before, so they have no way of coping with the anxiety that comes with meeting new people. In the case of the reader above, he jumped right into the deep end of the pool (a singles night), became terrified, ashamed of his reaction, and later questions his worth as a future romantic partner.

2. **They used to be an outgoing and personable guy, but the trauma of divorce left an emotional wound that is still in the process of healing.** These men are shocked at how going out to meet new people (something they used to be good at), or even something as simple as seeing a photo of a friend and their loving family is enough to trigger anxiety or even a full-blown panic attack. Men tend to underestimate their brokenness and attempt to overcome the obvious with false bravado and ego-driven stupidity. These guys just need to learn to walk again before they even think about running a marathon.

Most of the guys I talk to fall into one of the above two categories. Both need to take a time out, forget about jumping into the scary bottomless ocean, and instead go take some basic swimming lessons. They need to take very real and deliberate baby steps towards becoming a more centered and confident social person again. When you're a broken dude, people (especially women) can smell it a mile away. You may try to convince yourself that you're ready to jump in, but you'll end up breathing in water, panicking, and the lifeguard will have to jump in to save you. You'll be embarrassed and everyone will now see you as *"That guy that almost died"*. Not good.

Being social, like anything else, is a skill. It takes practice. It means being brave. It's being ok with being vulnerable around strangers. You achieve that state of social zen by gaining little wins along the way. How to start? Very simple. I like the plan of forcing yourself to talk to at least five people every day. Small talk, as we say in America. Nothing serious. You're not hitting on a girl. You're not trying to make best friends with some random guy. You're just putting yourself out there and saying, *"Hi. You don't know me… but here's something a little positive for you."*

Some ideas:

1. To some random guy at a parking lot: *"Dude. I love your car. What year is it? Very nice choice. Have a good one!"*

2. To some woman on an elevator: *"Those are some pretty snazzy boots. I like the leather. Very cool. Later!"*

3. To your waitress: *"Oh, the breakfast was very good. Thank you, Nancy. Don't work too hard today. Have a good one!"*

4. To a guy at work: *"Hey, thanks for that thing you did the other day. Much appreciated. I'm heading to the coffee shop. Want something? It's on me."*

5. To the old lady at the grocery store: *"Ma'am, do you need some*

help with that? Looks like a lot to carry."

Little positive steps. Makes the other person's day a little brighter. Makes you feel a little more positive, and with every interaction, a little braver and more confident. These quick positive interactions aren't anything like the scary singles event. At the singles event, you're just fumbling with your drink and staring at your shoes trying to get up the nerve to talk to the pretty brunette across the room. The reason that scenario is so stressful is because of the understood dynamic at play. You're looking for a mate, and so is she. That naturally means you're in a contest to win her over. You're competing with the dozens of other guys trying to get the hot chick's attention. Right away, the scenario is one of competition and pressure. She's judging you from the moment you step in the room. She may have made up her mind about you already, without saying a word to each other. Overall, it's just a bad scene for a socially awkward dude. You're introducing an unnecessarily high level of anxiety for absolutely no reason. If a singles function is your barometer for how you are doing socially, then you'll just fail and push yourself further into isolation and eventual depression.

You need little wins. The little wins build momentum. That's how you crawl out of your social anxiety hole. You do so by opening yourself up to people, making yourself a little vulnerable, adding a little something positive to the other person's day, and then backing off. The key to why these interactions are so genuine and effective is that there is no understood reciprocity at work. You just made them feel good, and you wanted nothing from them in return. With the singles event, there is always an expectation of return. If the woman agrees to talk to you, she is opening herself up to the very real possibility of being asked out, going on a horrible date, having to deal with a guy that she really doesn't like, turning him down for future dates, dealing with his emotions, etc. She has to give up a great deal of her time an energy to a probable lost cause and negative end result. To her, talking to some random nervous guy at a singles mixer is a big freaking deal. You, the nervous guy, may have already struck out and you don't even know it.

The singles mixer, online dating, meeting your friend's sister who recently got divorced… these all require next level social skills to navigate successfully. If you find yourself anxious around people, you need to get a lot of practice in before you jump into the deep end of the socializing pool.

The Secret to Picking Up Women

There are many expert "Pickup Artist" men out there that are willing to take a lot of your money to show you how to best attract women and get laid. Many socially awkward nice guys from all over the world regularly fork over thousands of bucks to go to boot camps and seminars run by former nerdy men who claim to have the secrets to unlocking physical and emotional intimacy from hot women. These programs are a mixture of human behavior study, evolutionary psychology, and motivational speaking. You can probably learn 99% of what they teach by doing YouTube searches and watching videos for a few days. It's nothing Earth-shattering. These Pickup Artists are simply nerdy guys who sat back and watched the Lover guys who so often succeed in getting laid and broke down their behaviors into digestible chunks of actionable behavior.

Allow me to save you a ton of time and money. I'll break it down the secrets for you:

1. Be attractive.
2. Be fun. Be different.
3. Be confident and aware of your value.

There… that's it. You're welcome. Now, let's break it down a little

94

further.

1. Be Attractive

Yes, it's important that you look good. Very important. Can't overstate it. I'm amazed at how many men don't realize how they LOOK has a great deal to do with why their ex-wife never seemed to want to have sex with him or why they can't seem to get a woman to return his messages. We're all animals, after all. We are all looking for certain indicators of physical health and virility. For women, they're looking for indicators of health, virility, and strength. Yes, they like muscles. I don't care what they tell you, they like muscles. They may not like giant balloon bodybuilder muscles. They may not like huge fat strongman muscles... but they like a guy who looks good in a t-shirt. They like a lean, mean fighting machine. They like a guy who can take care of himself AND take care of her in case things get sideways in a hurry. That want to be able to grab on to an arm or put a hand on your chest and feel something solid. They like a manly man.

They also like a man who looks like he cares about his appearance. They like a guy who keeps up with the fashion trends and doesn't look like he's stuck in the '80s. Put the jean shorts and white dad sneakers away. Get on a program like Menlo House that will send you hip and current clothing on a monthly basis. Basically, just act like you care about what you wear. Put some thought into it. How you decide to show yourself to the world is very important. Whether it's at the office, at the job site, at the singles bar... your clothes say it all. What are you saying? Are you saying, *"I'm a comfortable dad"* or are you saying, *"I'm fun and different from all the other guys my age. I'm actually pretty cool and interesting"*? The choice is yours.

2. Be Fun. Be Different.

"So, what do you like to do for fun?" This is the

quintessential dating ice-breaker for single women. What they are saying: *"So, tell me what life with you would be like."* If somebody today asks me that, I would say that I love working out, playing basketball, reading, writing, watching movies, going to sports games, art, playing guitar, and traveling to places like NYC, New Orleans, California, Costa Rica, Canada and Europe... oh, and I just started learning how to ski. That paints a pretty good picture of exactly WHO I am as a potential date. What if I said, *"I like fantasy football, craft beer, and golf"*? That says *"I do what every other guy out there does. There is absolutely NOTHING unique about me. Not a shred of mystery or fun here."* Zzzzzzzzz.

Be fun. Be different. Be INTERESTING. Stick out from the crowd. Think of what your dream date would say after spending a weekend with you. She's having coffee with her best friends and they ask, *"Soooo? How was the date with that guy you met online? What's he like?"* What's she going to say? *"Oh, he's nice. He has kids. Really good guy."* That's it? Wow. Before she can finish the sentence, she is thinking, *"Alright... maybe he's not that great after all. I'm wasting my time."* Remember, your dream date is a mentally healthy woman. That means she's got her shit together. She's not looking for a rock-solid father figure in her life. She's not looking for the guy who won't go anywhere when she acts crazy and breaks his stuff in a fit of rage. She's looking for the good guy that will be fun to be with. She's looking for the sexy diversion from her stressful life. Be THAT guy.

3. Be Confident and Aware of Abundance in Life.

If there's one thing that brings down good men in dating, it's the deep-down feeling that he is just not that great of a catch. His lack of self-worth makes it so that any and all attention he gets from women is to be cherished and held on to as long as humanly possible. He feels like he is LUCKY to get a reply back from a text he sends to a girl he met online. He is LUCKY to get a date with her. He is LUCKY to get a kiss from her. Never in the nice guy's wildest dreams does he ever feel that SHE is lucky to be in HIS presence. This state-of-mind permeates everything about his persona. Like sharks being able to smell a drop of blood a mile away, dangerous women can smell low self-esteem, vulnerability, and weakness just from something simple like your frequent text messages and self-deprecating humor.

You must always keep in mind that there are quite literally about 100,000 women that you are compatible with and they would date you and have a great time (assuming you have your shit together and are a man of value). I'm not going to tell you the typical, *"There are a million women out there for you!"* nonsense. Given geographical limitations and time, it's not THAT big of a pool of candidates, but it is a huge number that you're not ever going to exhaust. Trust me. The women are out there. Lots of them. Just the simple act of KNOWING that you have value and options in life already puts you above many men in the male dating pool. If you're out on a date with a woman and she instantly starts acting horrible and bluntly states that she's tired of dating losers who don't pay for everything… you can simply smile, shake her hand and say, *"Ha. I tell you what... I don't think this is going to work out"*. Then you walk away. You retain your self-respect, you save yourself from hours, days, months and possibly years of anguish at the hands of an awful woman… and you further set yourself apart from the crowd. Watch as the formerly angry woman eventually sends you text messages apologizing for her behavior.

She was in a bad mood. Work was terrible that day. She got into an argument with her sister. She was just not on her A game and she would like another chance. All of that may be true, but there's another side to the story: **You passed her test.** Yes, it was a test. She threw a proverbial punch at your face (her bitchy attitude) and you ducked and countered with right jab to her nose (your willingness to immediately walk away and forget her). You didn't stand there and take blow after blow from her. You're too tough and smart for that. You passed her test.

Women Test Men. Constantly.

If you sit back and watch people as I do, you start to notice certain behavioral dynamics come up again and again. Watch a single man and a single woman who are obviously attracted to each other meet for the first time at a party. They do the normal greetings we all do. He smiles to show he's healthy and has all his pearly white choppers. She shakes his hand... but not too roughly. She wants to come across as weak and submissive to his tougher masculine persona. She doesn't want to damage his fragile male ego. He sucks in his stomach to appear thinner. She starts twirling her hair and blushing slightly, both universal signs of arousal. Her red lipstick and makeup further give the impression of flushed skin. Yes, it's all one big, predictable, hilarious animalistic mating ritual.

Everything seems to be going well with the small talk, and then the woman decides to kick things up a notch. Almost out of nowhere, she will throw a test at him. This is commonly in the form of a very slight (or not so slight) insult. This may be some little verbal jab at an obvious fault of his (like his height or his age). It may be that she takes a piece of information the man just gave her and spins it around to make him look bad. *"My ex used to ride motorcycles, too. I have always thought of it as just a stupid mid-life crisis. There are so many other more worthwhile things to do if you want to enjoy life, in my opinion."*

With these female tests, there are a few ways to react:

1. **Explain, qualify and apologize.** In the case of the woman insulting his motorcycle hobby, the man may say, *"Yeah, I can totally see how you may think that. A lot of guys are poser dorks on the motorcycles. Lots of bored doctors and lawyers with too much*

money pretending to be bikers. I'm not like that at all, though. I take it very seriously. I don't know... I mean... maybe one day I'll grow tired of it and take up golf. Probably not a bad idea. Playing outlaw biker guy gets old after a while. My mom freaks out every time go for a ride. She's worried sick I will get in an accident. Hasn't happened yet, knock on wood."

With this reaction, the man just took his life's passion and completely threw it under the bus... all to appease the pretty woman he just met ten minutes ago. He instantly tried to explain and qualify himself by making fun of other men. This is a common ploy. *"I'm not like those OTHER guys!"* Then he brought up his mom, for some strange reason. Total swing and a miss. Instant loss of respect. She doesn't know why exactly, but she suddenly wants to go back and talk to that other guy she met earlier in the evening.

2. **Be insulted.** - *"Well, who asked you for your opinion, anyway? You know what, you're not all that, like you think you are. I'm wasting my time talking to you. Later."* If you're genuinely insulted and have no interest in the woman, this is certainly one direction to go in. Take what she says very seriously, let her know she angered you, and bail on the conversation. Keep in mind that what you feel may be a manly and "take no bullshit" way to walk away with your dignity may be seen by her and others as a major hissy fit from an overly-sensitive guy who lets a strange woman too easily dictate his mood. She played you like a puppet.

3. **Be playful and confident.** - *"Well, I was deeply involved in the world of male jello wrestling for many years, but I pulled a hamstring. Had to forfeit my championship belt. I got bored and I figured riding a bike was the next best thing. Don't get me wrong, I still break out the jello and baby pool on occasion. You know, for family BBQ's and stuff."* This reaction not only says, *"I have a sense of humor and don't take myself so seriously"*, but it also shows that

you are NOT affected on an emotional level by the random snotty comment by some gal you just met. You just don't take her seriously enough. Yes, she's pretty, but she's also just another human you met at a party. Big F'ing deal if she thinks bikes are stupid. She's not the Queen, and even if she was… you still wouldn't give a shit.

Yes, the female tests are very real, and they extend WAY beyond the dating phase of a relationship. Wives test their men up until the moment they're put in the ground (and probably after). Women have an innate need to measure and qualify important men in their life. The overall goal is to determine if you are worthy of their respect and their time. Respect and time are very limited in the world of the woman, and she can't mess around with somebody who will waste both (another way we could learn a thing or two from women). If you appear to be a really great guy, you're attractive enough and you click on an emotional level, BUT you immediately cave in to one little jab she throws your way, then you're immediately discarded and put in the *"Maybe I will date him when I need to talk and have a free meal"* pile… and for good reason: **You're weak**. You aren't ready for the dating game, and you're most certainly not worth her time.

A lot of men catch on to the tests that women put them through and will proudly proclaim that these are just GAMES women play, and they (as rational manly men) don't play games. Men like to feel that they are above the silly and shallow behavior that they see women putting men through. To that, I say:

"The game is going on whether you are playing or not. The entire mating ritual and subsequent relationship is one giant game."

From the moment you get up the nerve to approach the girl, to the birth of your first child, to the time you both retire, to the moment you take your last breath… the woman in your life is going to test the shit out of you. You may call it nagging, being a bitch, playing games, not saying what she really means, being deceitful, being manipulative, etc.… but it doesn't change the fact that it's all going on and it will absolutely continue to go on. You must recognize when the tests happen and know how to deal with them.

Here are some of the most common tests given by women in relationships:

Asking you to make a decision.

This is one that is the subject of countless internet memes and comedy routines. Wife says she is hungry. *"Where do you want to go eat?"* the husband asks. *"I don't know,"* wife says. Husband suggests Chinese food. Wife says no. Husband suggests pizza. Wife says no. And so on and so on. Husband gets frustrated. *"Just tell me what you feel like!"* For some reason, this makes the wife even more angry and frustrated. Husband interprets this as typical female indecision and a strange desire to make drama and chaos from something as innocuous as deciding where to go eat.

In this situation, the ideal (but rare) male response would be to say, *"Sweet. We're going for pizza. You have 10 minutes to get ready, Ms. Sexy Pants. If not ready by then, I'm going without you."* The wife may pout and act offended at his joking but abrasive attitude, but in the end, she will probably grab her stuff and go along and enjoy some pizza and have a little more respect for the man who can take charge and handle something as simple as where to go eat. Worst case is that she REALLY didn't feel like pizza that night and she will make sure to be a little more assertive next time and give her man some better direction. Win/Win. Respect and better communication in the end.

The question of where to eat sounds silly, but it really is a very good test of your ability to lead and make a decision and relieve her of that day-to-day stress that eats away at her attraction towards you. Simply put, indecisiveness on the part of the man is a sign of weakness. It means, *"Please don't give me the stress of making a decision. Please relieve me of this burden, oh mentally stronger woman in my life"*, or even worse, *"I'm afraid to give direction right now because I know you will just disagree with me and that makes me feel stressed and I can't take it so please just make the decision for us so that I know you are happy"*. Both are NOT good, and both result in a loss of respect.

"I saw you looking at that girl. Do you think she is cute?"

So many men cave into this test and approach it the wrong way. Remember as I said in chapter one, **"Why Did This Happen?"**, a woman's sexual attraction towards you depends on several factors, one of which is your ability to attract other women. If other women find you desirable, then your value as a partner just shot through the roof. If your woman flat out asks you if you find that other woman attractive, she's asking you if you are still an honest sexual being. Do you still have your very real and very normal sex drive that every healthy man should have? Are you willing to put up with your wife's possible shitty response and tell her the honest truth, or are you going to lie and tell her that you have zero attraction towards other obviously hot women in an effort to appease your wife's low self-esteem in that brief moment?

The right answer is a form of playful honesty. *"Yeah, she's not bad. I sure wouldn't kick her out of bed"* or *"What? I'm sorry, I didn't hear what you said. I was fantasizing about life with that 19-year-old that just walked past us."* These responses show that you are honest and playful, but also that a pretty girl walking by and getting your attention is no big deal. It happens all the time. Nothing to freak out about. What you don't do is explain away and tell her that no other woman exists and that she is crazy for thinking you are staring at some obviously pretty girl. Of course you were staring at the girl. Your WIFE was staring at the girl.

Everyone in the vicinity was staring at her. It was a pretty girl. That's like saying, *"DON'T STARE AT THE BEAUTIFUL SUNSET!"* You're going to stare. It's completely natural. So, man up and be honest. Deal with the subsequent hissy fit from your wife, and deal with the long-term positive repercussions of a wife who respects you a little more for being an honest man with a healthy libido.

"Are you saying you'd rather go out with your friends instead of being with me?"

As men, we like to get away from women on a regular basis and recalibrate our sense of self. We like our time with our buddies or time alone to ourselves. This is normal and healthy. This is why guys like to go to the garage to tinker with the car, escape to the "man cave" to play some guitar, hang out and play poker with the boys, etc. All of those things do NOT involve the women in our lives. It keeps us mentally balanced. This is an understood part of being a man and one a sane and healthy partner would recognize and support.

When your woman has a fit of low self-esteem or anxiety about your relationship and asks, *"What… you don't want to be with me on Saturday? You'd rather go hang out with Dave and drink beer and watch football?"*, she is seeing if you NEED her (neediness is not good) and will chicken out and cave in to her emotions (fear of her is not good). The answer from any man should be, *"Yes, of course. I enjoy time with my friends. It's good for me. I will see you on Sunday. Love you, babe."* If your woman takes great offense to this and you honestly feel that she always NEEDS to be with you, then you should probably question the long-term viability of your relationship. She is exhibiting an inability to cope with the stress of being alone and may have a very real fear of abandonment. These are two signs that your world is about to go right down the shitter in a hurry. You've been warned.

"Please put up a boundary for me and save me from my own bad decision-making."

I saved the best for last. As far as common woman tests are concerned, this is the one that is one of the most insidious. Your wife may very well be right at the edge of crossing the line into inappropriate behavior territory, and she has either consciously or subconsciously reached out to you for help. She wants you to play the bad guy, figuratively smack her on the behind and say, *"No! Bad girl!"*

An example of this may be, *"Do you feel bad when I go out drinking with my friends on Fridays? I know I've been out the past three weeks and left you with the kids. I don't want you to be mad."* (a common scenario discussed earlier). So many men respond to this in the complete wrong way. *"No! Baby, seriously. Go out and have fun! I love when you enjoy yourself. The kids and I are fine."* Usually, the man is NOT fine with such an arrangement, but he doesn't want to rock the boat and have a pissy wife sitting at home pouting on a Friday. Plus, his nice guy ways make him recoil at the thought of playing the part of the bad guy. He always wants to be Mr. Agreeable Guy. In his mind, that's the more secure and honorable method of being a husband.

Even if the man were in fact completely okay with his wife going out on the town four Fridays in a row (maybe he likes the time alone to mentally recalibrate), the mere act of his wife bringing it up and asking his opinion should cause his gut to question the reality of the situation. Why is she asking him this now? Probably because she recognizes that her behavior is coming close to crossing the line and she's a little scared of what may happen next… yet she, for whatever reason, feels powerless to stop it herself. Maybe she heavily flirted with several guys at the dance club last week and can't wait to go back and do it again. Maybe she drank way too much and got sick and felt like a bad mom, yet she can't imagine a boring Friday at home with her husband and kids.

104

Whatever the case may be, by approaching the man and saying *"Are you SURE this is okay with you?"*, she's, in essence, saying, *"Please show me your invested enough in us as a couple that you don't mind playing the bad guy and telling me to act like a responsible adult."* When the man says, *"No, everything is cool"*, the wife's internal response is, *"Oh well. I tried. I guess he doesn't care."* Yes, it's childish. Remember, it's all just a big stupid game.

Show her you care. Show her you don't mind playing the bad guy. Show her you don't mind the inevitable fit that will come your way. You are in the relationship for the long haul, and many times that means playing a paternal role that many men just aren't comfortable with. As with all these tests, show her you don't mind putting on the Captain's uniform and leading. There's nothing sexier than a man in a uniform, even if it's a metaphorical one.

The Delicate Balancing Game

Let's face it, being in a relationship is being a man on hard mode. It's a constant struggle of maintaining your independence, compromising when appropriate, validating, being sensitive, vulnerable, tough, stoic, honest and true to your sexuality… all at the same time. It's learning when you're being tested, when you need to apologize, and when you just need to shut the hell up and walk away from the situation temporarily… or maybe even permanently.

The walk away part is what is toughest for nice guys. Broken women that are in relationships with nice guys understand this better than anyone. They know they can get away with murder. If you give them an inch, they will absolutely take a mile. They can say and do what they want with impunity. These are the women that will kick a man when he is down. They recognize that they can push and cross over boundaries regularly and the nice guy will always give them the benefit of the doubt. The MHNNM, on the other hand, always has the "walk away forever" card in his back pocket, and he's not afraid to use it. He's not afraid to be the biggest asshole on the planet Earth for the few minutes it takes to say, *"I think I'm done with us. I appreciate all you've done, but this is over."*

The winner in all relationships (professional, platonic, or romantic) is the one that has the least to lose. He or she can walk away and say, "It's cool. No biggy. Have a great life." The loser is the one that absolutely NEEDS the relationship to continue or else their whole life falls apart. The users and manipulators pick up on this NEED and take full advantage of it. The guy at the office who has no backbone, no marketable skills, and no other job prospects is asked again and again to come in on weekends and stay late to finish up some projects. The guy who knows how to play office politics and has a good network of professional connections gets to play golf and drink beers with the boss instead. He knows how to play the game. He found the right balance for the relationship.

A man needs to find the right balance between nice/sensitive and tough/stoic for his romantic relationships. You have to wear both the Lover and the Provider hats. Many men fresh out of bad relationships will recognize that they stayed too long on the nice/sensitive (Provider) side of the fence and watched as it slowly eroded away at the health of his relationship. In response, his post-relationship self will swing that pendulum all the way over to the other side and attempt to become a super alpha male tough guy. He's the one that can be heard saying, *"All women are whores"* after a few beers with his buddies. He's the one that will stomp his feet and yell *"Well, fuck you, you slut!"* after being turned down by a woman at the dance club. He's simply pissed that he's not invited to the fun relationship party. He thought he played by the rules (by being a nice guy) and life didn't reward him as he thought it should. So, he tries out plan B: **Embracing his asshole side.** What a lot of guys unfortunately realize is that there are many women out there who actually DO prefer being intimate with a selfish mean asshole over a pushover nice guy. If the former nice guy turns into an asshole and starts getting laid a lot more… he's going to remain an asshole for quite a while. In fact, he may even turn the asshole dial up a few notches. As far as he's concerned, it works. Then he gets hurt in some way, and he goes back to the comfort of the typical nice guy routine again.

The secret, like all things in life, is in the middle ground. It's remaining stoic in your approach to stress that life (and your wife) throws at you, being a ruthless bastard when you need to be, and randomly doing nice things for your woman just because you love her to death and you want her to feel appreciated for all that she does for you and your family. It's also being willing and able to play the part of the ultimate bad guy and walking away from it all when the negatives far outweigh the positives.

Is the Juice Worth the Squeeze?

There's a time in every relationship where a man looks at the constant struggle of maintaining the delicate balance of Lover/Provider and he asks himself, *"Is it worth it?"* Is dealing with her constant tests and nagging worth the once a week great sex and close friendship? Are her beautiful smile and fantastic backside enough to overcome her near-constant fits of angry jealousy? Do her great qualities as a mom and friend overcome her expanding waistline and her lack of sex drive? Does he grow tired of having to constantly play the paternal role and keeping his wife from crossing the line into inappropriate behavior territory? Does he just wish she would grow up and stop being so damn emotional half the time?

"Show me the hottest woman on the planet, and I'll show you a guy that is sick of her shit."

For the MHNNM who is trying out a monogamous relationship, his patience may be razor thin. After all, he recognizes the abundance of casual relationship candidates that are out there, he recognizes his value as a mate, the value of his time, and he recognizes the potential danger involved with some of the glaring red flags that others would simply write off as "typical girlfriend behavior".

To the MHNNM, having a casual girlfriend who constantly questions his whereabouts is not worth the hassle. He knows potentially dangerous abandonment issues when he sees them. A woman who always seems to be trying to make him jealous will be dropped quicker than she can say, *"A cute guy at the gym today said I was really hot and wanted my number"*. The MHNNM recognizes unhealthy attention-seeking habits. He just has no time or patience for the silliness. Could he be dropping genuinely good long-term relationship candidates by bailing out so quickly? Is he far too impatient? Maybe. Maybe not. Again, the MHNNM doesn't NEED a long-term relationship to function, so he can afford to let a good one slip through the cracks if that means dropping twelves other psychos that could ruin the life he has worked so hard for. Ironically, his willingness to hit the eject button makes him way more attractive. Remember, women want what they can't have. If he's not chasing, then his value must be high.

For some men in long-term relationships, these *"Is it all worth it?"* questions are eventually answered for them when they have an affair with the cute 20-year-old from work and leave their wife and family. That's the easy and chickenshit way out of a difficult situation. They hit the restart button with a new fresh face and ride off into the sunset as the intense high of the new relationship floods their brain. As a guy once told me years ago, *"Man... there ain't nothing better in the world than new pussy."* The man who runs off with his new girlfriend will eventually just do the whole long relationship process all over again. First the new relationship energy with tons of sex. Then the familiarity. Back to boredom. Back to drama. The resignation. Rinse and repeat.

For most men, however, they linger in a state of relationship limbo for years. They're not quite happy with several parts of the relationship, but they convince themselves that they are happy enough with the other parts. They make do with what they have. They don't want to rock the boat and potentially ruin the whole marriage just because they're not happy with several huge negative things their wife does on a regular basis.

For the nice guy that avoids confrontation and just "lets it go" on a regular basis, he's actually telling his wife that their relationship isn't worth the hard work needed to make it better. More specifically, SHE isn't worth the hard work. SHE isn't worth being honest with and telling her when she is doing something that is slowly but surely eating away at his attraction to her. Instead, the nice guy will put up with his wife's negative actions, ignore, and occasionally physically and mentally escape from her. The wife will eventually pick up on his growing resentment. She may see that he is becoming more distant and disconnected from her and ask him what is wrong. The man, on the other hand, feels that his wife should just KNOW when she's doing something wrong. He shouldn't HAVE to tell her (a very feminine quality of the nice guy). Eventually, the resentment and anger may boil over, usually at a very stressful time, and the husband blows up at the wife. The wife sits back and listens. Instead of apologizing or empathizing with her husband's feelings, she is instead overwhelmed by her disgust with him in that moment. Why? Because he had issues with her over all these months/years, and he was too scared to tell her. *"Wow... what kind of man is he?"* All of this drama could've been avoided if the man just took a chance months or years ago and said, *"Stop. What you're doing right now is not good. I don't like it."* When he finally blows his top, the wife's subsequent lack of empathy and remorse is baffling and further infuriating to the man. The resentment continues to build for both partners.

Once you are in a committed relationship with a woman,

109

you have to decide if the inevitable hard work of keeping the relationship machine running is really worth the time and effort. If you see so many red flags and your foreseeable future is filled with abuse or unnecessary stress, then you need to take the next step and do what is right for both you and her. End the relationship. But, before doing so, ask yourself what part YOU played in bringing about the current situation. Did you do all you could to improve yourself and the relationship? Have you really been the captain of the ship and played the role necessary to keep the boat afloat? Have you truly stepped up and been the fearless asshole that you sometimes need to be? More often than not, the answer is no. Live and learn.

Your current relationship may be over for good, but you need to take the right energy and the right mindset into your future. If you're like most men I work with, you will end up with another woman… probably sooner than you realize. The rush of positive energy that a seemingly "perfect" woman brings to your world is beyond intoxicating. Before you know it, your bank account is drained, you're taking care of somebody else's kid, and you're wondering why it burns when you pee.

Be very careful.

PART TWO
YOU NEED A MISSION

Goals. Hobbies. A daily checklist. You need something that keeps your inner fire burning. You need to work towards something meaningful. You need positive momentum, or you absolutely will stagnate. If your wife and kids were your sole mission in life, you were doing it all wrong. You need to be a complete man with something else to strive for.

It's time to get off your ass and do something different.

Chapter 4: Keep Busy

Are you having trouble getting over your ex? Still feel like she's "the one" and no other woman on the planet can possibly come close to earning the love you feel for her? Can't conceive of a life without her? All of this is totally understandable. Make no mistake about it, you are mentally and physically addicted to your wife. She has been in your little world for YEARS and every facet of your life has her stamp on it. From your daily routine, your kids, vacations, etc... she was there. She's another limb on your body. For that to suddenly GO AWAY is not a little thing. It's nothing short of traumatic.

Just like when trying to break an addiction to a drug such as alcohol, getting over your ex is a really difficult thing to do. Your body and brain will be saying, *"Now, hold on a second. Wait... Let's talk about this first."* Unfortunately, there is no magic bullet cure for getting over your ex in a hurry. You can't take medication to make all the pain go away and never return. Getting over a lost love is a slow and gradual process that you can either expedite or make it drag on for YEARS. I have talked to men who have literally watched their ex have multiple affairs, divorce him, remarry, divorce again, remarry again... and yet they STILL have feelings for her and dream of getting back together. Why? Because they're still addicted. They are still taking the occasional shot of the ex-wife whiskey instead of putting the bottle down and stopping cold turkey. They're still hanging around the proverbial bar on Fridays. They didn't do the really hard but necessary work of breaking that bond. If they did, they would be looking at that woman with the extreme disdain and eventual indifference that she deserves and not daydreaming about one day getting back together.

If there's one piece of advice I give to EVERY man trying to get over a failed relationship, it's to **"KEEP BUSY".** For the sake of your sanity, your overall health and your future on this planet, you absolutely must have things to do. This is the work needed to move on in life and break the bond with your ex. You need goals to work towards. You need to accomplish things. No, you cannot just do your normal day-to-day routine of work, come home, collapse on the couch, drink beer, and fall asleep. You need to put down on paper what you want to accomplish, outline the steps to accomplish these goals, and check them off as you go. When complete, you move on to the next goal. You do this again, and again and again. You accomplish things. Lots of things. That's called living.

A recent article on the website of Psychology Today talked about a phenomenon that was coined by researches at UCLA studying depression: **"Empty Man Syndrome"**. To quote the article:

"On one of my first days there, I heard my colleagues whispering about a patient. One mumbled something about 'empty' that I couldn't quite hear. I jumped into the conversation and asked what they were talking about. She replied, 'I said he has 'Empty-man syndrome'.' Intrigued, I asked her what that was. It was a term she came up with to describe certain men with depression. It applies to guys in their 40s and up who were single or divorced, and don't have any friends, are unemployed or stuck in a job they don't like and have no real hobbies. I asked why she came up with a term for this, and she sighed, 'Because they don't ever seem to get better.'"

Men get depressed. It happens quite a bit. Thanks to our innate need to provide and protect our loved ones, we can very easily allow the mundane nature of our work and parenting life to get in the way of doing all the other things we need to do to keep our brain and body healthy. We all know the dad who works a ton of hours and comes home and collapses and does it all over again the next day. You may have even been that guy. If you don't exercise both your mind and your body in the way that is right for you, they will both atrophy. Being in a marriage and having kids tends to gradually accomplish this negative spiral for many men.

There are two important things that every man needs in order to avoid the slippery slope of chronic depression:

1. **Social Support.** As much as I say you don't NEED to have real love or marriage to be a complete man, you DO need to have some type of regular social contact and support network in place. You need family, friends, and loved ones that are there for you in times of need. You need consistent human contact in a meaningful way. Socialization is a basic human need. This is why solitary confinement is considered an inhumane form of punishment by many. It literally drives you crazy.

2. **Feeling like you have a purpose in life.** This one is especially true for men after their marriage dissolves. Men often use their marriage/kids/family as their sole purpose in life, so to suddenly yank that away is absolutely horrible and life-questioning. Many alcohol, drug, and food problems start when men hit rock bottom after divorce. When you have no purpose in life, you will fill the void with something… and it's usually nothing good.

Being more social and finding a purpose (or multiple purposes) are not insurmountable tasks. Most of the time you can accomplish both via the action of going out and DOING things. You need to take action. You need to build momentum. You have to take the first step, then another step, and so on. Once you get up and get going, it's amazing what you can accomplish. I know better than anyone, that first step is the toughest. The good news is that the first step is simply using your brain and asking yourself, *"Okay… what is it that I WANT?"*

For most men, they have an inkling of what it is they

115

WANT to do, but it's a matter of actually putting together the plan, and incrementally taking the steps necessary to accomplish the goal. The good news is that accomplishing these goals also puts you in touch with a growing circle of new friends and loved ones that help you along the way. It's a win-win situation. It's just a matter of kicking yourself in the butt and getting started.

Choosing Your Mission

Get out a pen and paper. It's time to write down a list. I want you to throw aside all of your preconceptions about what you have the time to do. Pretend you have all the time and energy in the world. Get yourself in a child-like mindset of adventure and possibilities. Don't worry about anyone judging you. Your nag of an ex-wife isn't here. Your mom and dad don't need to know about this. Forget what you buddies might think. Keep it to yourself.

Now, write down a list of the things you like and want to do. Could be things you already do from time to time, or it could be things you always wanted to do. Here's an example of a list you could write down. Just play pretend and go along with it for now.

1. Join a gym.
2. Gardening.
3. Remodeling the house.
4. Rebuilding old cars.
5. Learning to fly a drone and take aerial photos.
6. Skiing.
7. Scuba diving.
8. Ballroom dancing.
9. Getting a pilot's license.
10. Learn archery.

Those are just ten things that came off the top of my head. It's a collection of the different things I have heard men and friends say over the years. Some of these items may seem a little more "out there" or more unobtainable than others. Maybe you're like many divorced men and time and money are both not easy to come by right now and that affects your short-term goals. That's totally understandable.

Look at your list and put a star next to those items that can be started right away. You need some quick wins under your belt. We don't want to get bogged down in details of the goals that aren't realistic until five years from now. The big dream stuff is great, and they are on your list for a reason, but we can't tackle them right now. For me personally, I would say learning to fly a plane would NOT be a realistic goal for me at this time in my life. I have too many other things going on and getting my pilot's license takes many hours and lots of money that I simply don't have. Scuba diving lessons? Not going to happen anytime soon. There is an indoor scuba school about an hour from here that I could go to and take classes, but that's not high on my list of must-do things. Scuba diving is a skill I may use once or twice from now until the day I die. Maybe one day I'll look into it, but not right now. Not a big deal. Instead, for me, I would put a star next to going to the gym, gardening, and ballroom dancing.

Now that you have put a star next to those realistic and attainable goals/activities, it's time to put a plan of action into place. First, prioritize what you have starred on the list. If three of your items are starred, take a look at those and rank them according to what lights your fire. Which one really makes you say, *"Yeah... That would be really fun and interesting."* That is your number one priority right now. We are tackling just one thing at a time. Again... we're after some quick wins.

You now need to put together a set of steps needed to get started and to also maintain the hobby/goal/activity. For example, if I really wanted to learn ballroom dancing (I know... just go with it), the steps would be:

1. Research classes. Pick a school.
2. Set time to go take a lesson.
3. Attend a lesson.
4. Go every single week for the next three months, no matter what.

What's going to happen after you climb off the couch and attend classes during those three months? You will meet new people. Probably a lot of women. Women are more social creatures, after all, so they are usually the first ones to sign up for any new group activities or classes. You will probably be one of the few men in the class. You will meet an all-around different group of adventurous adults who all had the same idea you had: *"It might be kinda cool to learn how to dance like I've seen on TV"*. They're all in the same boat. They're in the class to better themselves and enjoy life. When you surround yourself with such positive and outgoing people, your perspective on life starts to change. You become more energized. Momentum builds. Somebody in the class that you became friends with suggests that you should also try out a yoga class with them. They've been going for a few weeks and it's amazing. Their back has never felt better… oh and the chicks in their yoga class make the ballroom dancers look like a nursing home!

Next thing you know, you're now in a yoga class once a week, staring at young in-shape women sweating in tights. You suddenly love yoga. Now you regularly attend both a dance and a yoga class that you weren't taking before. After a few weeks, you decide to give yoga a three month trial as well. You enjoy ballroom dancing so much that you're going to keep it going past the three-month period, at least until the teacher says you're good enough to leave or maybe graduate to a different class. With those two classes going on every week, you'll notice the pounds start to melt off. Your agility and cardio capacity go way up. Flexibility is way up. You're just all around healthier and more vibrant. You enjoy the classes so much that you don't groan and belly ache over having to go. You sometimes even throw in an extra class here and there if time allows. Positive momentum is building. You find yourself trying to recruit friends and family to join you.

Now that you've added those two activities to your regular weekly schedule, they don't feel like extra work. They just simply replaced the pointless TV time or the time you spent playing Xbox and watching porn. Now you start thinking about the NEXT step. You want to add something else to the mix. The positive snowball is building. Once you get going and you get some "wins" under your belt, it's hard to stop the progress. It just happens. Then the end of the year comes, and you look back and say, *"Damn. I got a lot of shit done."*

Be In Control

Whatever your mission may be, there needs to be an overall theme of "taking control" of your life. You need to throw out all of the "woe is me" notions of **life doing things to you.** Hey, life always presents you with very real obstacles and very real opportunities. That's just what life does. You can make all the plans you want, but life may decide is has something else entirely in store for you. **"Man plans and God laughs".** Sometimes it seems like the stupid obstacles way outnumber any positive opportunities you may have in the foreseeable future. It sometimes may even seem overwhelmingly negative, to the point of being one big cosmic joke. The car breaks down, the dishwasher leaks all over the kitchen, you stepped in dog shit on your way to work, your boss tells you you're getting laid off, and your wife suddenly wants a divorce. Hey, it happens… so how do you respond? Do you look at the cards you are dealt and figure out how play them, or do you throw your cards down on the table and pout about what a shitty hand you have? Which option do you think will generate actual results and a way

119

out of the shitstorm of problems?

It amazes me how many men go on and on about their life situation as if they are telling me about a new novel they are reading. They talk about themselves almost in the third person. They're detached. Out of control. Helpless. Sometimes they are frozen by indecisiveness. Sometimes they KNOW exactly what they need to do next, but it's just too damn hard and they are too damn tired. They have zero momentum. They need some help.

You need to take a moment and "look down" on yourself from above. Take a good long look at yourself from an outsider's objective point of view. If you're a religious person, maybe it helps to put yourself in God's shoes for a moment. If you're a science fiction guy, maybe look at you and your life as one big computer simulation. You're in a giant video game of life. When you are presented with all this overwhelmingly negative bullshit in life, it's like meeting the video game "boss" at the end of the level. Do you throw down the controller and say "fuck it" because beating the boss is seemingly impossible? Do you start all over at the beginning and get to the boss again and try out a different strategy? Maybe you should go on the internet and look for a cheat code that will give you unlimited firepower so you can breeze through the boss and make it to the next level. Whatever the solution is, there IS a solution there. Sometimes it's just a matter of picking up the damn controller and getting to work. Make the little guy (you) jump over the fire, climb up on the moving platform, grab the golden key, beat the dragon, and save the princess.

You gotta take control. Today. Move forward. DO SOMETHING. Get help if you need it. Your future self will thank you.

Chapter 5: Mandatory Mission #1: Your Body

Okay, let's set aside the imaginary world of ballroom dancing and yoga for now. I used those two examples because they illustrate how you can really step outside of your comfort zone, leave the house, attend some classes, use your body in new ways, and mingle with a new and successful group of people. For many of you, going to a class like that just ain't gonna happen. You could be working two jobs and have three kids to watch full time. You could live out in the middle of nowhere and Walmart is the only sign of civilization within 50 miles of you. Maybe the closest thing to yoga in your area is watching the town drunks collapse in awkward positions at the public park. Hey, I grew up in the middle of nowhere America.

Let's think about what you CAN do right now. Remember, your final to-do list should be realistic and attainable. You need some wins under your belt. You need to build up some real and serious momentum. There is one subject that should always be at or near the top of your mission list. It's the one thing that you have absolutely ZERO excuses to ignore. It's the one thing you walk around with every single day, 24/7. It's the one thing you probably have ignored far too much over the years. We're talking about your body. Simply put, you need to get your ass in shape and take care of yourself. Your BODY should be your #1 mission in life. The good news is that building up your body and improving your health will probably be the most rewarding mission you've ever been on.

All missions are deemed worthwhile and sustainable when you achieve something along the way. If you decided you wanted to write a book (like I'm doing right now), you get started typing away at your computer, maybe not even caring about the outline or organization of your book at first. Along the way, you check the total word count, stop and read sections out loud… and you smile. *"I'm actually doing this. I'm going to be an author when it's all said and done. How cool is that?"* As you progress, the organization of the book takes shape. Chapters begin to form. Paragraphs are moved around. Sections are deleted. Thoughts come to you out of thin air. *"Serendipity"*, they call it. You're in a state of flow. Hours fly by like minutes.

When you decide to take on your body as a mission, you start seeing results pretty quickly. Eating right and exercising just makes you feel and look a lot better. The pants are looser. The shirts fit better. The blood pressure goes down. You're able to walk up 20 flights of stairs with no problem. You can lift up your kids like they're nothing. Each little moment is a step towards building momentum. Next thing you know, you're at the Mexican restaurant telling your kids to keep the basket of chips the hell away from you and you're ordering the grilled chicken dinner. You can't wait to hit the next physical milestone, and a dumb basket of salty tortilla chips isn't going to stop you from getting there. You are a man on a mission.

Sleep

I put this first for a reason. Men, most of you are chronically sleep-deprived. You are not getting the amount of sleep that you need to be at your best level physically and mentally. It's time that we set aside our antiquated notions of staying up late at night watching TV with a beer in hand and getting up at the crack of dawn to tackle our work day. Getting up early is fine, as long as you get to bed early, too. Don't think that working on less than eight hours of sleep per day somehow makes you more a more productive man. In fact, it does just the opposite.

You need sleep to rebuild both your brain and your body. Think of sleep as the time your body says, *"Okay, we have some much-needed cleaning and repairs to do, and we need you to pass out while we do it."* If you're routinely cutting back on your sleep, below the scientifically-proven threshold of eight hours, you're in essence interrupting that important cleaning and rebuilding process. Some important stuff will be left undone. When you wake up too early, the little janitors and repairmen running around in your body and brain throw their tools down in disgust. *"Well, I guess once again I'm not mopping the bathroom floor! This is going to get really gross in a hurry if I don't get to do my job!"*

We know for a fact that lack of adequate sleep puts you at risk for the following:

- Heart disease
- High blood pressure
- Diabetes
- Lower sex drive
- Depression
- Weight gain
- Advanced aging
- Memory loss
- Increased risk of Alzheimers

If you routinely sleep less than six to seven hours per night, you increase your risk of cancer by 50%.

Getting sleep is no joke. The days of bragging about getting by on five hours of shut-eye are long gone. Thanks to science, we now know what a horrible idea that is. Feeling groggy at 2:00 pm every? Get a quick nap in. Do whatever you can to shut your eyes for 20 minutes. Sneak away from your office if you have to. Your body needs that rebuilding time. You will be a more productive human if you listen to your body and get the rest it NEEDS to properly function.

Get your butt to bed early. Your life depends on it.

You Are What You Eat

Contrary to what many people may think, if you really want to make yourself look and feel better, a good 90% of the necessary work revolves around your diet. As fitness gurus will tell you: *"Abs start in the kitchen"*. You can work your tail off in the gym, bench press the equivalent of a small elephant, sweat so much you could fill a baby pool, and you can very quickly erase ALL of that hard work with a diet of pizza, chips, and beer. The muscle you worked so hard to build will be hidden under a thick layer of blubber. The guy who works 1/4 as much as you do in the gym but eats a healthy diet will look better and will be a lot healthier than your fat-but-strong self.

I can't tell you how many guys I see at the gym that bust their butt on a regular basis and have absolutely nothing to show for it. For YEARS they look the same. Sure, their bench press and deadlift gradually go up (something they will undoubtedly tell everyone within earshot about), but as far as people outside of the gym and his own doctor are concerned, he's the woefully out-of-shape fat guy who is one pizza slice away from a stroke. He could do a complete 180 change if he simply stopped shoving crap in his piehole. The strong guy at the gym that looks like a sumo wrestler is probably just six to twelve months of healthy eating away from turning heads and looking like a legit "holy shit" lean muscular guy with abs that everyone admires.

To keep it brief: **Stop putting unhealthy shit into your body.** Don't complicate this. Don't play dumb. You KNOW what the "unhealthy shit" is. It's not rocket science. Stop bullshitting yourself and everyone around you.

It's easy to SAY, but it's not necessarily easy to DO. The lure of unhealthy food is incredibly strong. That crap is literally engineered to appeal to your mouth and your brain and cause you to eat more and more and more. The snack companies have this stuff down to a science. Everything from the proper amount of

124

sweet and saltiness, to the mouthfeel and crunch. It's been tested again and again until they get it just right. Then they put it on the market and rake in the millions as the world gets more obese and Type 2 Diabetes and heart disease kill us by the thousands. They're drug pushers, basically, and we're all their loyal junkies.

Hey, don't get me wrong… I love snacks. They're freaking amazing. Salty crunchy crap is my heroin. Put a giant bowl of Chex Mix in front of me, and that bastard is decimated in minutes. That's why I can't have it in the house. I don't buy chips. No pretzels. No crackers. No deliciously perfect Chex Mix. If they were here, they would be gone in no time That's my own personal boundary I have to put up to keep my health in check. You see, I get fat easily. I'm not some flawless fitness Adonis here. I'm a fat guy in an in-shape guy's body. It takes a lot of work for me to stay in shape. Is it worth it? Hell yeah. What's the alternative? It's not a pretty sight. Trust me.

Think about a horribly out-of-shape 50-year-old fat dude with oxygen tubes in his nose sitting in a doctor's office listening to a concerned doctor tell him about the dangers of congestive heart failure and how he needs to go on eight different medications and probably get his stomach stapled or else he's going to die. Think that guy is sitting there saying, *"Yeah, but doc… those pizzas and beer were fucking awesome!"*? No. The poor slob is thinking, *"What have I done? I don't want to die like this. Jesus Christ, what a waste of a life."* If you're a young guy, take it from older guys like me… 50 will be here TOMORROW. The years just fly by. You don't want to waste that precious time and ruin your golden years because something tasted really good and made you feel happy for five minutes. You're not some bored housewife crying while shoving ice cream in your face and chasing it down with a bottle of wine. **You're a man. Act like one. Put the cupcakes down.**

I'm telling you, if you simply start eating like a guy who cares about his health… you're going to feel and look a thousand times better. If you combine healthy eating with a regular, rigorous exercise program, the sky is the limit on just how good you can look and feel. A whole new world will open up to you.

What Diet is Right for You?

The problem for a lot of guys that decide to get in shape is that the fitness world, as a whole, is so damn confusing. There are literally hundreds of diet and fitness plans out there. There are vegetarian diets, all-meat diets, ketogenic diets, high carb diets… you name it, and somebody has "proof" that their way of eating is the absolute best possible way, period. My opinion? Well, I just go by what the science tells us, and it's pretty simple:

The only successful diet is one that YOU can maintain over a long period of time.

That's it. If that means a ketogenic diet of meats and greens and very low to no carbs works best for you AND you actually enjoy it with no major urges for carbs and no cheating… congrats, you found your meal plan for life (yes, for life). Maybe you find that a Mediterranean Diet is more up your alley. Maybe you have personal reasons to go vegetarian. Maybe you learn that you need a cheat meal just once a week to keep you sane and active. Maybe you eat a very strict diet during the week and workout like an animal so you can get away with an entire cheat day of sweets and pizza every Saturday and your waistline stays small and your health doesn't suffer (lucky you).

Every person is different. If you're on a meal plan that has you regularly crashing and binge-eating junk food, gaining five pounds, and then starting over again to try and lose that five pounds… and then do it over again… only to end up gaining 12 pounds after 12 months, well then you are not on the right meal plan for you. That will not work out for you, long-term. You're setting yourself up for catastrophic failure and a myriad of health problems. Time for Plan B. What is Plan B? No idea. I'm not you. That's up to you to test out and see what works best for you and your body and lifestyle. But first, you need to do the work of determining what your current starting point is and go from there. Click here to see my own personal diet.

Get Thee to a Doctor

Prior to any kind of diet change, I highly recommend you go to the doc and get a full workup done. Check out your blood lipids, your thyroid, and your hormone levels. If your thyroid levels are out of whack and your testosterone is at the level of a 90 year old man (more common than you may think), you may need to begin taking medications that will get you to a baseline "normal" level before starting on your healthy journey. You can do a super strict healthy diet and work your ass off in the gym five days a week, but if your total testosterone is 120 (when it should be closer to 1,000), then you are just going to be beating your head against the wall in frustration. You'll follow a plan for months and just end up looking like dog shit. Then you'll switch plans. Then the new plan won't work, either. Then you'll give up. You'll go back to eating crap and skipping the gym, and you'll be worse off than you were before. If you're going to do something, do it right. Go get checked out by your doc as soon as possible.

At the time of this writing (early 2019), there is a bit of a medical/fitness renaissance going on as it pertains to unique individual preventative care and fitness. What we're learning goes beyond simply saying, "everyone is different". Thanks to relatively inexpensive at-home DNA testing companies like 23andMe.com, you can spit into a vial, send it in the mail, and a short time later get a detailed report telling you everything about yourself from your ancestry to your predisposition to specific diseases and disorders. It's absolutely ground-breaking for personal health and fitness. The concept of "guesswork" and a "one system is best for everyone" is going right out the window.

I personally used a combination of 23andMe.com and DNAfit.com to learn that I have genes that suggest I am very carb intolerant, a slow metabolizer of caffeine, intolerant of booze/marijuana, and I'm especially sensitive to salt. I don't need as much vitamin D as I thought I did, I need to watch eating too much charred/smoked meats, and I need to eat more cruciferous veggies. I also need to up my intake of vitamin A, C, and B12. Workout wise, I am more inclined to do best at endurance sports (a shock to me…a longtime weight trainer) and I have the capacity for a high VO2 max (the amount of oxygen I can use during intense exercise). I also have a higher likelihood of injury from working out.

As the science gets better, information about my own specific DNA profile will continue to trickle in. On a regular basis, I get reports showing my likelihood of type 2 diabetes, dementia, macular degeneration, etc. I find it all to be extremely interesting and can't wait to see what advancements in the DNA world take place over the next ten years. Soon we will be able to completely tailor our diet and fitness regimen to fit our specific individual needs and limitations. No longer will we ask our in-shape buddy, "So, what kind of workout should I do? How about my diet?" You'll know exactly what YOU need to do to look good and live as long and as healthy as possible. It may be a completely different prescription compared to your buddy.

Testosterone Replacement Therapy

If you've read my website, you know that I am on Testosterone Replacement Therapy (TRT). I inject an oil-based compounded testosterone solution into my butt twice a week, every week. I've been on this regimen for over five years now. It works well for me. It takes me to a physical and mental state that I otherwise would not be in. Does that make me less of a man? Meh… maybe. With every shot I take, I'm admitting that I am not a natural badass. I'm a guy who found out he had a deficiency, took meds and felt better. It's no different than a person who takes any other kind of medication to bring them to a baseline level of health.

There is a strange stigma around TRT. There's an obvious level of scrutiny and shaming that you don't see with other "wellness" therapies. Why? Because we're talking about treating men. If I was a woman going to the doctor and saying, *"I would like to stop my periods because they are heavy and very painful"* or just simply, *"I would like to go on some form of birth control so that I can have sex worry-free",* the doctor would give me a literal menu of choices to choose from, and all will drastically alter my hormonal makeup. I could take a shot every few months, pills every day, implants, etc. Are there dangers to these drugs? Of course. Some of the dangers can be pretty significant. So then why are the doctors so eager and willing to prescribe these drugs? Simply put, the freedom to manipulate your body as you see fit and to take control of your own fertility is seen as an empowering statement of female freedom in an otherwise oppressive society. The woman finally gets to control what goes on with her body. With every pill she swallows, she is saying, *"I'M in charge of ME."*

I cannot be overstated: **The advent of the birth control pill dramatically changed the sexual landscape in the western world, and the medical industry hasn't looked back since.** If you're a doctor and a female patient comes to you wanting to go on birth control, you don't question her motivations. You would never in a million years say, **"Why? You're supposed to be making babies, young lady. You're a woman. That's what you do. Pills aren't really natural, anyway. They can be dangerous. Have you tried condoms? If you must do birth control, that's the way to go."** You'd be out of a job faster than you can say #metoo.

Now, pretend for a moment that you go to the doctor and ask for a blood test so that you can see where your testosterone levels are. The first thing the doc says: *"Why?"* You explain that you're getting older and you have certain symptoms that are concerning you. You list the symptoms and show the doc the data that shows that they could be alleviated by reaching proper levels of testosterone. You just want to see where your levels are at right now. The doctor chuckles. *"These are all perfectly natural things you're experiencing. Welcome to getting older. If you find that you are depressed, I can certainly put you on an SSRI. There are also some great therapists in the area you can talk to."* If you push further on the matter, the doc may get a bit hostile. You're not only questioning his authority, but you're also now one of THOSE guys. You will hear how not everyone is a He-Man and you just need to accept your lot in life. Plus, there are numerous dangers around testosterone therapy. They will tell you about prostate cancer, heart attacks, strokes, etc. Then he will pat you on the back and chuckle as he motions you out of his office. *"Let me know if you want to try out Prozac. I have many patients on it with wonderful results."*

Many doctors throw mind-altering (and arguably dangerous) substances like SSRI's, and even opioids at their patients like they are parade candy but go ahead and ask about testosterone… and watch your doctor's mood abruptly change. You immediately go from being a regular boring patient to some dumb guy having a midlife crisis. Why is that, exactly? Why is it that even a guy who has done a ton of homework, brings literature to his doctor, and asks for a simple blood test laughed at and dismissed so quickly? I think it's primarily a sexist attitude. *"Not everyone is a He-Man"* your doc may bluntly tell you. It's a not-so-nice way of saying, *"Know your place in society. Go tend to your kids, change diapers and sit at a desk all day. Being manly is best left to the real men who don't need a shot in the butt."*

In short, when it comes to men, nobody likes an imposter. Society wants the real thing. We want a natural. The second that somebody picks up on you TRYING to be more "manly" (being fake) they will turn on you. You will be blatantly laughed at by the very people you trust with your health… and probably even by your close family and friends. Not unexpectedly, these are also the same people that will dissuade you from all forms of self-improvement. They like you in the comfortable boring Provider role that you are in. If you suddenly want to switch things up and change your role, they will pull every trick in the book to keep you where you are. More often than not, the first thing they go to is using shame to manipulate you.

I'm not going to tell you that TRT is right for you. I'm no doctor. All I can tell you is my own personal experience:

- I gained muscle
- I lost body fat
- Lowered anxiety/stress
- I feel more confident

Have there been negative side effects? Yes. For one, I have learned that I need to control my estrogen levels via an additional medication called Arimidex. To oversimplify the science behind it, your body may try to counteract the higher testosterone levels you are introducing by increasing the opposing hormone known as estrogen. This is done by the aromatase enzyme, via a process in the body called aromatization. To counteract this, you can take an aromatase inhibitor (AI) like Arimidex (there are other types and brands of AI medications). Not everyone on TRT needs an AI, but I did. Without it, I would bloat and grow breasts. Seriously. But, if I take too much AI, it will lower my estrogen to levels that are way too low and I will experience joint pain, emotional flatness, lowered libido and an increased chance of heart disease. Luckily, I have learned how to avoid this with proper minimal dosages.

Overall, my experience with TRT has been positive. Since I've been on, my blood pressure has not gone up, my cholesterol levels are fine, and my hormonal levels are within balance. One thing that did creep up was my red blood cell count. To alleviate that, I make sure I drink a lot of water and I donate blood. Problem solved.

Two more negatives to consider when on testosterone:

1. **You are on it for life.** This isn't a "one shot and you're cured" kind of deal. This is a regular regimen of taking your shot (or applying your cream) every single week for the rest of your life. Oh, sure, you can stop your TRT at any time, but your body will go back down to testosterone levels lower than they were before, and it may take additional drugs to help restart your body's natural production again (HCG, for example). You'll eventually be back at your low baseline level and feel like crap all over again. Many men don't last long at this stage. Once you have felt "normal" or better, you don't want to go back.

2. **Fertility will most likely be lowered or gone completely.** Trying to have a kid? Plan to have any in the near future? Do yourself a favor and go get some of your sperm frozen and stored. Go to the fertility clinic, run a few batches, and put that baby batter on ice. It will cost a small fortune, but you'll have to do it if you want to have kids in the future AND be on testosterone. Why? The little secret that nobody likes to tell you is that testosterone is a potent form of birth control for most men. By introducing an external source of testosterone to the body, your testes will shut down their own production… and subsequently the production of sperm. It's your body's way of saying, "*I see I'm getting my testosterone from an outside source now. Welp, no need for these testicles anymore.*" Yes, your balls may atrophy and shrink down in size. This can be alleviated by taking a compound known as HCG (another shot). Even while on HCG and sporting a full set of testicles, most men report that their sperm count as at or near zero.

132

In short, if you want to get a woman pregnant, you probably need to be off of testosterone or have some potent sperm ready to thaw out.

Working Out

Ninety percent of how you look and feel may be determined by your diet and sleep, but the remaining 10% is built by working out. Training. Sweating. Hitting the gym. Busting your ass. Doing it repeatedly. Pushing yourself. Going for a walk is fine and dandy (and very good for you), but it's not working out. It's not busting your ass. That's what old sedentary people do after their doc puts them on blood pressure meds and recommends they move instead of sitting all day long. "Working out" goes beyond that. We're talking about training yourself. It means shocking your body so that it is forced to build muscle and lose body fat. It's going to mean stepping outside of your comfort zone in a big way. It's also a shit ton of fun and changes your life in so many ways.

For you guys with limited funds and time, the good news is that the gym is not needed to gain that extra 10%. It's great to have access to a large number of weights and machines to sculpt your physique, but you can attain a fantastic level of fitness by doing bodyweight exercises in your bedroom. Push-ups, burpees, dips, yoga, squats, lunges, jumping… all of these are ready to do right this minute. You just need a floor and your body. That's it. Want to kick it up a notch? Go online and order a jump rope, a kettlebell or two, some bands, and a medicine ball. Now you have another twelve months' worth of exercises you can do before you get bored and need something more advanced.

I could go on and on about an exact workout routine, but I won't bother. There are so many out there. Just like diet, you need one that is right for you… and one that you will maintain consistently over a long period of time (with positive results). My recommendation is to mix things up. Do various things to keep it interesting and keep the body guessing: Military-style calisthenics, bodybuilding-style weight training, steady state cardio, high-intensity interval training, powerlifting, martial arts, gymnastics, yoga… the list goes on and on. Pick what you like. Do it. Then do it again. Consistently. Have fun with it. If it gets stale, try something else out.

Yes, you can overdo it. "Overtraining" is real, especially for you older guys out there. You want to look forward to going to the gym or doing your home workout. You want to approach this mission with energy and joy. You don't want to feel so sore that you need three days of rest to recover. You don't want to start breaking your body down and getting sore throats and cold chills the day after your workout. That's your immune system telling you to cut it out and back off. You want to sleep, eat and drink enough to provide the fuel you need to hit your workouts with motivation and positive energy.

For my personality type, I tend to REALLY get into a new hobby/interest and go as hard as I can, get burned out, and move on to something else. Working out is no different. If I walk into the gym, I want to see how much weight I can lift and try to squeeeeeze out that last repetition until I reach the point of absolute failure. Then I move on to the next exercise and do it again. Three sets… gradually increasing the weight… absolute failure. Then on to the next exercise. That plan worked when I was younger. I put on some good muscle that way when I was in my 20's. Now… that would be a quick way to injury and absolute certain burnout. Now I need to tell myself to hold back a little. I usually finish a workout set well short of my absolute failure. Now when I do an exercise, I concentrate on feeling the muscles work. I focus on my form and proper range of motion. I finish my sets with some gas left in the tank. I take a breather, gather myself, get a drink of water, and then continue on with my workout. My workouts are usually around an hour to an hour and a half long and do I feel drained… but in a good way. I don't feel like I've been hit by a truck. My muscles feel full, my head feels clearer, my clothes are drenched, and I'm ready to tackle the rest of my day. That's the state of zen you want to be in as a result of working out.

Again, I'm not going to tell YOU what to do to build YOUR body. Use Google to come up with different workout ideas. YouTube has an endless number of videos. AthleanX is a great program if you want to spend some money. Maybe find a good trainer to help you out. Maybe go to one of the many garage-style gyms that are popping up all over the place. They usually have a prescribed plan in place and a series of stations set up for people to do. You go around and complete each station at your own pace (with the guidance of a coach). It's usually a good combination of cardio, high-intensity interval training, and lifting weights. My wife goes to such a gym (along with two different yoga classes). She loves it, and she's not a natural gym-goer by any means. She likes that she is told what to do, she does it, she gets better each time, and her body thanks her for it. That's what you want to do… find a program that helps you achieve the little important wins along the way. Like with anything in life, the momentum is key. You need to move forward in a positive direction on a regular basis. The end result will be a completely new you looking back at yourself in the mirror.

Do it. Your life will change immensely. Personal health and fitness are the building blocks of a foundation for a good life. Once you have that sturdy foundation, everything else just seems to click in place.

Here is an example week of working out for me. I like to mix things up to keep from getting bored, so the following week may be completely different. Google these exercises if you're not familiar with them:

Monday: 30 Minutes Stair Master, Dumbbell Bench Press, Dips, Tricep Pull-Downs, Face Pulls, Dumbbell Pullovers, Battle Ropes, Abs, Stretches

Tuesday: 30 Minutes Eliptical, Wide Grip Pull-Downs, Hammer Strength Rows, Straight Arm Pull-Downs, Barbell Curls, Kettle Bell Swings, Abs, Stretches

Wednesday: Stretches, Light Yoga, Basketball

Thursday: 30 Minutes Stair Master, Leg Presses, Leg Extensions, Glute Work with Bands, Hamstring Curls, Kettle Bell Swings, Stretches, Abs

Friday: Stretches, Light Yoga, Basketball

Saturday: 30 Minutes Eliptical, Standing Dumbbell Shoulder Press, Dumbbell Laterals, Face Pulls, Kettle Bell Clean and Press, Abs, Stretches

Sunday: Rest

Note that I like to throw in a healthy amount of cardio to start off my workout days. First, it's good for me and my heart. Second, it gets my body warmed up and better prepared for weights. Third, it burns calories. Fourth, I just feel better overall when I do cardio. I DO NOT enjoy it. It bores me to tears. That's why I have my headphones in and listen to podcasts, type ideas into my phone as they come to me, read stuff online… whatever to pass the time.

You'll also note that I follow the old bodybuilding workout style of "body splits". I concentrate on chest and triceps one day, then back and biceps another day, shoulders, legs, etc. I tend to not mix them up in one workout. It's just something I've grown accustomed to and I have no scientific basis for doing so. I just like concentrating on building and maintaining specific parts of my body and then resting and focusing on another part the next day. Works for me. You may like more infrequent total-body workouts. Totally up to you. Both styles produce results.

Trying to Lose Fat? Be patient.

Losing body fat is a tricky thing. For those that are morbidly obese, they tend to see the biggest results within the shortest time frame. Take a 500 lb. guy and put him on a healthy diet and exercise program, and he could easily lose 10 lbs. per week. After all, it takes a lot of work for a 500 lb. guy to maintain that huge unhealthy shape. It takes lots and lots of eating high-calorie foods over a long period of time. It's not an easy job. Take away the excess food, and get them moving in new ways, and their body sighs in relief and starts melting away the fat cells. *"Finally, I can stop being so damn fat. That really sucked."*

On the other hand, take a muscular 200 lb. guy at 16% body fat who works out regularly, but he would really like to be 185 lbs. at 8% body fat. That is a whole different story. His body wants to maintain those 200 lbs and will do all it can to stay there. If you're in that boat, BE PATIENT. A half-pound or a pound a week of weight loss is not bad at all. Keep it up and you'll see results, but it will be extremely tough. You will have to work A LOT harder and a lot smarter to get to that "unnatural" level of lean muscularity. As Lyle McDonald outlines in his book **"The Stubborn Fat Solution"**, the fat loss can sometimes seem to happen in "whooshes". You'll be eating at a deficit, working hard in the gym, and yet you notice the numbers on the scale go up two pounds. It makes no sense! Why bother working so hard? Then a short few days later you'll notice you've lost four pounds. You gained two, but then you lost four… net loss of two pounds. Why did this happen? Well, it may very well be your body increasing water retention in an effort to maintain weight… and then finally giving up and letting go of the water and some of those stubborn fat cells. I've personally noticed this phenomenon in my own body. I'm not a gradual fat loser. My weight loss stalls, and then the fat and water whooshes off in bursts. I've gone to bed and woken up a different person.

Want to look like those fitness models you see in the ads? Be aware of what you're getting yourself into. The use of anabolic steroids and other chemicals for burning fat and maintaining muscle is extremely common in the world of modeling. Those abs and veins you see online and in the magazines aren't "natural". That is an extreme state for the body to be in, and typically they're in that shape for a very short amount of time. Yes, the models are naturally gifted athletic people who look a whole lot better than most of us, but that extreme level of muscularity and low body fat that is you see in the ads for supplements and exercise equipment is not an easy and normal state for them to maintain. Those people use whatever edge they can to achieve that "whoa" effect for the day of the photo shoot, and then they go back to their normal non-depleted state. Don't fall into the trap of comparing yourself to others, especially when the game is not a level playing field and what you're seeing is not at all realistic. You just work on being the best YOU possible.

Be realistic about your goals. Put your health first. Work hard, eat right, stay positive… and you'll be rewarded when you look in the mirror.

Chapter 6: Mandatory Mission #2: Your Money

I've been broke. It sucks. It drains you of what little life energy you have left. The burden of debt and bills piling up weighs heavily on your shoulders 24/7. You could have the greatest day ever, and it's ruined by a letter from your credit card company letting you know that your rate has just been bumped to 27% due to untimely payments. Then your boss lays you off. Then the alternator goes out on your piece of shit car. Throw kids in the mix… and good luck. It sucks. Boy, does it suck.

They say money can't buy you happiness…and they're right, but it sure as hell helps get you there quicker. Having money gives you options in life you simply don't have when you're broke. Having money means NOT having to do something to make a few bucks just so you can pay your gas bill. Having money means dealing with the busted alternator like the minor annoyance that it should be. Being flush with cash means having "fuck you" money when your boss wants you to do something unethical or he wants you to work 80 hours a week with no pay raise. You simply walk away from a bad and unhealthy situation. If you have a pile of money saved up and no debt, you can take your time and find a better job.

Money = Freedom.

For some divorced men, they watch half (or more) of their freedom-giving money go right into the pockets of attorneys and the ex-wife. Alimony and child support can absolutely wreck a man. It could be that you're now saddled with half of the total family debt (even though most was not yours… I speak from experience). You can go from a big beautiful house with a garage and man cave, to a tiny apartment with a mold problem, thin walls, and neighbors that have loud sex at 3:00 am. Tell THAT guy that money can't buy him happiness.

As far as basic "must do" missions are concerned, your money should come right after your body. Like getting in shape, getting your money problems resolved is NOT impossible. It may take a good amount of time. It may, at times, seem insurmountable. It may take a lot of uncomfortable work. But... it's doable and it's well worth it. When you have both your health and your finances in order, the positive momentum train starts going at an unbelievably fast pace. Things start clicking for you. The snowball builds and builds. It's amazing what you can accomplish when the weight of the world is off your shoulders (and off your stomach).

You must treat your money situation in the same way you treat all of your other life missions. You TAKE CONTROL. You don't let it control you. One step at a time. Check items off your list as you go. Yes, it's true that money, like food, has a strong emotional component tied to it. You feel absolutely amazing when you buy the $35k new car with the leather seats and all the fancy doodads inside. Your rational brain would tell you to buy the high mileage but reliable $10k car instead and pocket the $25k extra in payments and invest it (or use it to pay off debts). After time, you can eventually turn that $25k into $50k or more. Instead, the irrational and pleasure-seeking side of your brain convinces you that the extra $25k you spent on the car was well worth it. You DESERVE the fancier car, you tell yourself. It has that awesome huge sunroof and the heated seats! The navigation! The rear-facing camera! Next thing you know, you find yourself signing a lengthy contract for making large monthly payments over an extended period of time... for a rapidly depreciating asset. The moment you drive that shiny new car off the lot, it's worth less than when you saw first took it for a test drive. That's not a "smart" investment, but it's an understandable and emotional purchase. That emotion is what you need to recognize while it's happening and take control of if you want to achieve financial freedom.

Money is just simple math. To conquer it, you MUST remove emotion from the equation.

Beware of Manic Optimism

Divorce is an understandably emotional time for everyone. For some men in an acute state of mental distress, this time of "starting over" can lead to a series of life-changing mistakes that just further complicates their lives and makes everything exponentially worse. You'll hear about the guy whose wife left him and then he suddenly started questioning everything in his world. His whole life up to this point flashes before his eyes, and it all seems like such a soul-sucking waste. Why on Earth did he work so hard and for so long when it just resulted in such an unhappy ending? He played by the book of rules, and he got shafted in the worst way possible.

The poor sap surprises all his friends and family when he decides to take his career and job in a new direction. Usually, this involves some kind of entrepreneurial endeavor. The betrayed man now feels that life is too short to waste at his soul-sucking insurance job for one more day, and he just quits out of the blue. If that wasn't enough, he then sells everything he has to buy equipment to follow his dreams of fixing up old cars. It's almost as if this new trauma he is enduring has spring-boarded into an early mid-life crisis. Ironically, everyone notices the similarities to his ex-wife. *"Oh man. First Sally went nuts and had an affair... and now Jim is quitting his job and acting crazy. Those poor kids."*

In no time at all, the man is dead broke and his ex-wife now has full custody of the kids. The overly optimistic and emotion-driven side of him took hold and set him back even further on his quest to start over. He eventually crawls back to his insurance job with his tail between his legs, along with several new tattoos.

There's a very common and temporary state of manic optimism that some men in crisis situations go through. All those things that they say they didn't have "the balls" to do earlier in life now suddenly seem more attainable. Fixing up old cars for a living doesn't sound far fetched when your boundaries and common

141

sense are broken down by trauma. You convince yourself that the kids will be "fine", you can still make your rent payments, and you can put food on the table. You just need to sell some things and maybe get your buddies to help you out with some loans… besides, you're going to be so awesome at restoring old cars that your bank account will be fatter than ever! You'll be able to buy your next house in cash! Unfortunately, that reality rarely, if ever, pans out. The vast majority of entrepreneurial dreams fail.

Chasing a passion and using it to make cash is a great thing. Quitting your regular-paying job and saying "to hell with everything" with no alternative plan or direction in mind is not so smart. Nearly 100% of people in such scenarios fail. It's at times like these when you should harness that energy and the "rebuilding high" you may be on and direct it in a more thoughtful and rational manner. Chasing a dream is awesome but do so in a manner that is well thought out, planned and takes into account scenarios for very real failure. In other words, **don't quit your day job**. If you have a lifelong passion that is calling you, and if you want it bad enough, then you will absolutely find a way to scratch that itch and still maintain your day-to-day obligations. You will find time to learn and pursue your dream. If that means working two jobs seven days a week to do it, then that's what it means. If you want the dream bad enough, you'll do the hard work necessary to keep your delicate post-divorce life machine running as smoothly as possible.

Don't let the overwhelming emotion of the moment cloud your judgment and lead you down a road you can't come back from.

Embrace Your Male Cheapness

A lot of men will tell me that even though more than half their family income left with their ex-wife, it eventually starts to feel like they got a big pay raise. Why is that? Well, the fact is that **women spend 85% of household income**. They may not make

85% of the family's money, but they still manage to spend it. If something is needed for the home, for the kids, for herself, or even for the man in the house… more often than not it's the woman going to the store or shopping online. This is why the term "Chief Purchasing Office" has been coined to describe the woman's role in the family.

If we're being completely honest, the majority of the spending done is very emotional in nature. The wife may be absolutely convinced that she needs the $2,200 red rug for the living room, instead of the cheaper one from Home Depot that costs $250. She'll give you a thousand reasons why the red one is the better choice. You end up getting the red rug (happy wife/happy life). All of your wife's rationalizing goes out the window when the dog takes a nice runny shit on the fancy new red rug the first day you put it down. Suddenly, the wife verbalizes how it would be nice to have the extra $2,000 in the bank right now instead of a red rug with a permanent discoloration thanks to Fifi the chihuahua.

Men typically look at things like a new rug and right away say to themselves, *"Do I NEED it?"* The answer, understandably, is NO. There's no NEED for those extra fancy things like expensive red rugs, so they are put off for another day (like when they get a wife). Recently, a tweet by a young woman went viral on the internet. In the tweet, she posted an image of a typical bland, spartan man apartment with a TV and a recliner in the living room… and that was it. In her tweet, she said, *"Guys really live in apartments like this and don't see any issue."* Yep, we sure do. When my wife and I met, I had a plastic storage container flipped upside down next to my bed. That was my bedside table. I didn't give two shits about how ridiculous it looked. I was a divorced dad of three kids and had a pile of bills to contend with. I just needed something to put a lamp and alarm clock on. Going shopping for a bedside table was never even on my radar. My house was a place to sleep, eat, shower and take a dump. My home was not a fashion statement or an attempt to impress anyone. It was shelter. The more spartan I kept it, the less I had to take care of and the more money I could put towards my debts and bills. Sorry if that made me less attractive, but my bank account really didn't give a shit.

Men with "fuck you" money don't go out and buy expensive bedside tables or $2,200 red rugs for their dog to shit on. Men with "fuck you" money see what their bank account really is: basic math. They buy what they need, get themselves the occasional toy, take care of the kids' needs, pay the damn bills, and they SAVE. You can call it being "cheap". You can call it being "frugal". You can say it's *"typical boring man behavior"*. Whatever you call it, it's your number one weapon to achieving financial independence. Embrace your boring, rational, masculine cheapness, because it will absolutely save your butt in your new post-divorce life.

Yes, I admit, 90% of the nice things we have in our house right now wouldn't be here if it wasn't for my wife. The place looks amazing. I'm glad that she has the eye for decorating and such things. I'm grateful that she's generous enough to buy a lot of these things for us. It makes for a beautiful place to come home to. It makes it our home. But for a newly-divorced guy who is starting over in life, the world of decorating and prettifying your home for the sake of impressing others is the last thing you need right now. Let the ladies handle that (and no, you don't need a lady right now, either).

Some quick facts:

$7 trillion in consumer and business spending is contributed by women in the U.S.

2/3 of the consumer wealth in America will belong to women within the next decade.

85% of purchases and purchase influences are made by women.

50% of products marketed to men are purchased by women.

60% of all personal wealth in American is held by women.

51% of all stock in America is held by women.

92% of vacations are purchased by women.

93% of food is purchased by women.

Over the course of a family's life, 90% of married women will control its wealth.

Now you see why the government freaks out about our rapidly decreasing marriage and birth rates. Without a woman in the picture, this whole marriage-based economy of ours falls flat on its face. Try to imagine for a moment a neighborhood of just single men. That would be one boring place with nothing but "good enough" houses with spartan furniture inside and guys hanging out playing video games, fiddling with guitars and fixing cars in the driveway.

Get Out of Debt

Debt is crippling. Debt is the gorilla sitting on your shoulders waiting to smack you upside the head and take a giant shit on you every time you feel like you have made some kind of financial progress. Your boss gives you a 10% raise, but your credit card interest just shot up to 27% due to a late payment. Ouch.

That's debt.

You have to get out of debt. The faster the better. You can't make substantial progress towards a better life with a dark cloud

145

of debt hanging over you. Car payments, credit card payments, personal loans, etc.… They are not good for you and for your future.

There is a popular plan for paying off debt called the "debt snowball". It was coined by radio personality and entrepreneur Dave Ramsey. Dave's show is a mix of religious conservatism and old-fashioned financial advice. It's a wildly popular and syndicated show heard on over 600 radio stations across the U.S. It is the third most popular talk radio show today. People seem to have a real hunger for improving their financial shape.

The essence of the debt snowball is simple:

1. List your debts smallest to largest.

2. Put whatever you can towards paying off the smallest debt first. Forget about interest rates. Continue making minimum payments on all the other, larger debts while you throw money at debt #1.

3. Once that smallest debt is paid off, take whatever money you were putting towards the small debt and now apply it towards the next largest debt, on top of the minimum payment you were already making.

4. Continue this down the line of debts until everything is paid off.

That is the debt snowball. Yes, it works. I know, for some of you smart-at-math types, you want to tackle the higher interest debts first. It makes more sense to tackle the $5k debt with 26% interest than the $500 debt with 1% interest. The point of tackling the small debt first is purely psychological. If you achieve the quick win of paying off the small debt first, you build momentum and you're better able to tackle the rest of your debts with the positive energy you will need. Getting out of debt is a tough hill to climb, so you'll need all the positive energy and momentum you can get. It's very easy to get discouraged and just "live with" making unnecessary payments for the rest of your life.

The Cost of Marriage

Thanks to our natural desire to provide for and protect our loved ones, we often find that our money situation starts going downhill fast the moment we fall in love with a woman. You buy gifts. You go on that romantic couples trip she's been talking about. You chip in for gifts for her friend's wedding. You buy a nicer car (to impress her). You buy nicer clothes (to impress her). Her friend has a baby shower, so you have to buy a gift. Not just any gift, though. You can't look cheap compared to her other friends. Then she needs help fixing her car that she damaged when she backed into that telephone pole. Then there's an awesome sale at the mall for underwear that she promises she will model for you. Then it's her birthday. Christmas time! Next thing you know, you're sitting down with your boss saying, *"So... is there any way I can get a raise?"*

Then, you get married. You quickly learn that marriage is a giant money-producing machine for a lot of different industries, and you're the ATM. Simply stated, marriage keeps our consumer economy rolling along. First, it starts with the way-overpriced ring, the wedding itself (the venue, food, decorations, dresses, tuxes, etc), the honeymoon, the expensive house, the cars, all the expensive stuff that goes in the house... the spending never seems to stop. And then... you have kids. Holy shit, kids are expensive. Nothing compares to the expense of having children. It really makes me cringe when I hear people say that you shouldn't think about silly things like money when it comes to having kids. You should just let nature take its course. People just want to pop out little snot-noses and give zero thought as to how they will pay for them. They'll spend hours researching the right SUV to buy, but creating a new human being is left up to our animalistic urges and biochemistry. Your wife wants a kid? Time to make a kid. Forget about the impact on your life and just procreate, dammit!

Years ago, a close friend of mine and his wife were expecting their first child. He was asking me about the various aspects of being a dad, including the all-important costs involved. He was a very frugal man. To him, money was basic math. He already saw thousands of dollars going out the door in his pre-kid married life, and he wanted to know what other surprises were in store for him. *"So, I've researched a lot about how much kids cost on average. I read where each one is about $200k over their life. Does that sound right?"* I just looked at him and laughed. *"How much do you have? Whatever it is, they will find a way to spend it."*

Take Advantage of This Time

Divorce is a giant financial reset button for many men. You have effectively eliminated the biggest factor that impacts your family's spending habits: **Your wife.** This is not demonizing all women. I'm not saying they are financially-irresponsible nutbags who whip out their credit card every five seconds. This is just highlighting the reality: For good or bad, **women spend the vast majority of dollars in the family, and men tend to not spend if they don't absolutely have to** (I know, there are exceptions to the rule). Take advantage of this time. Stay away from women for a while and get your finances in order. You've been given a financial time out. Use it wisely.

Get out of debt. Save. Invest. Get help if you need it. Make a giant game out of it. That's exactly what it is. See your money as a scoreboard. Keep spreadsheets tracking where you're at financially. Watch as the debt slowly goes down and the savings slowly goes up. Sell stuff you don't need. Do side gigs for extra income. Use the internet. Buy and flip things on eBay. Work your ass off on the job and ask for a raise. Your single biggest tool for getting yourself in better financial shape is your income. For many men, a 10% raise would change their life. Go get it. Then do it again. Then go get a better job. One step at a time. TAKE CONTROL of your finances.

Chapter 7: Obstacles

Other than the obvious hard work, dedication, and discipline needed to complete your goals and missions in life, there are more not-so-obvious obstacles in the way of you becoming the man you're truly capable of. You thought this was going to be easy?

The people in your life, at times, will seem to want to do all they can to stop you from becoming a better YOU. They will express concern, they will shame, and they will sabotage your efforts to improve. Again, this is just human nature. Some of it is well-intentioned, but some of it is the **petty and immature projection of their own failings in life.** Most of the people getting in the way of your success will be those closest to you. Some of the hardest work you will have to do will be to step over and around them without alienating them completely. Sometimes that is impossible, and the only proper course of action is to remove them from your life. This is one of the toughest things a typical nice guy can do in life, but it is so very worth it, as every successful person will tell you. Life is short, and there is no room for toxic people on your road to happiness and fulfillment.

The Well-Intentioned Worriers

Here's a very real-world scenario: Your little sister loves talking about you to her friends and neighbors whenever she gets the chance. If you're at a social gathering with her, she will quickly grab you by the arm and bring you over to her friends, as if showing off her prize possession. *"This is George, he's my big bro I was telling you guys about!"* What's she so happy and about? Why is she so proud? Her big bro is the nicest and sweetest guy on the planet Earth, of course. He's good with his kids, he's good with his siblings, he's good to his wife, and he's a really hard worker. She hopes to one day land a guy just like her big brother.

Your sister is closing in on 30 years of age, and she's growing tired of the conga line of *"cute but not husband material"* idiots that she meets online. After several one-night stands, lots of "ghosting" and a few failed short-term relationships, your sister is more than a little pissed about the quality of the male dating pool available today. She considers her big brother to be the beacon of hope for women like her. Yes, nice and sweet family guys still exist amongst the sea of dipshits losers she meets on a regular basis.

When little sister learns about your marriage breaking up, she is just as heartbroken as you are. Your ex becomes her sworn enemy for life. She will bad-mouth that woman at every opportunity. She seeths with anger when the topic of your divorce comes up. Doesn't that dumb cow of a woman realize what a perfect guy she had!? How dare she hurt her big brother like this! *"Don't worry"*, she tells you over coffee one day. *"You'll find somebody else. There are a million women looking for a guy like you. Trust me. I know from experience."*

You take your sister's words to heart and feel extremely optimistic, even excited, about the world of dating that lies ahead of you. All of the other women in your life say much of the same thing as your sister: You will have NO problem finding a nice girl who is looking for somebody just like you. You're a diamond in the rough. *"Trust me"*, they all say. *"You'll have ZERO trouble."*

The problem? You quickly learn that they are all wrong.

You play the sweet nice guy game for a while and get nowhere. Lots of expensive dates. Lots of dinners. Lots of pecks on the cheek and "good night" as the women go back to their apartments and don't invite you in. Your long texting conversations with the cute gals from Match.com go on for hours, but they come to an abrupt stop when you decide to escalate and sway them towards the topic of actually going on a date. You're a great buddy to many women you meet, but not *"boyfriend material"*, as one of your more honest female friends tells you. She's right. Going beyond the buddy phase is proving to be nearly impossible.

CHAPTER 7: OBSTACLES

Then you get frustrated and start looking for advice. You come across books like this one, listen to some friends who have luck with women, or just naturally become a more selfish guy who's no longer so hung up on finding a woman. You have other missions and goals in life and decide to focus on them instead. Unbelievably, the sex life kicks into overdrive. You can't believe it yourself, sometimes. By not caring so much about dating, by focusing on yourself and by not looking for the next Mrs. Right, you're able to meet your intimacy needs… and then some. That's when your sister wakes up, notices what you've been up to, and changes her tune.

Little sis doesn't like what she sees. She notices that you've lost weight, dress differently, drive a different car, and she saw you out with three different women over the past couple of months. It doesn't take long until she puts two and two together. You've become one of those asshole "player" types that she meets again and again on Tinder and Match.com. *"Oh no… not my perfect teddy bear of a brother!"*

Little sister is the perfect example of a well-intentioned loving friend or family member that holds you up on the pedestal of being a really super nice person. They believe that we live in a world of selfishness and shallowness and it's nice to know that there are good people like you still out there. What they don't see is that you routinely get stepped on, taken advantage of, and sometimes abused all in the name of being a "nice guy". Ironically, people like your little sister repeatedly demonstrate through their own actions just how wrong they are about relationships in general. They really don't know a damn thing about the modern-day mating game as their lack of a real and loving relationship so obviously demonstrates.

Your sister is not alone in her worries. Your best friend Dustin and his wife are concerned, too. Dustin says you need to stop with dating around and meeting all these women for sex. He thinks you need to just grow up and go back to the old you. He

153

sees value in settling down and working on a family. He sees what you are doing as "giving up" on the dream. He tries to set you up with a single mom he knows who has four kids of her own. She's been unlucky in the dating department. She's vocal about finding a great guy to settle down with. You politely decline. This really pisses Dustin off. *"You can't go on pretending to be Mr. Playboy forever. Eventually, you're going to want to marry again and it will be too late."* It's obvious that his wife's female-centric point-of-view (time is a factor and you must marry) has now infected your buddy's perspective.

You listen to his concerns because he is your best friend and he means well, but Dustin's attitude starts getting on your damn nerves. You eventually reach the end of your rope and point out the obvious giant elephant in the room: **He's not in a happy marriage.** Not at all. Of all your married friends, Dustin is probably the most miserable and the biggest stereotypical Provider of them all. You let him have it. *"Oh yeah? How's that working out for you, exactly? Didn't you tell me that you two haven't had sex in months, your wife won't give you blowjobs, and all she does is complain about being fat and show she hates her body? Weren't you caught looking at porn not once, not twice, but three times? Didn't she get so pissed that she bought you a book about porn addiction? Isn't that what you just told me a couple of weeks ago when you came over for beers? Why in the hell would I dive headfirst back into that life? Been there, done that, got the divorce to prove it. I'm going to take my time and get shit straight in my life for once. I'm not going to force a relationship just so I can be back in the same boat again."*

The well-intentioned worriers are always oblivious to their own faults. Your overweight mom is worried about your "drastic weight loss" and tries to get you to eat more. Your promiscuous sister who routinely turns down nice guys doesn't want you to be a Lover like all the other guys she meets and gladly gives sex to. Your sexless best friend who hates his boring life says you should also just give up on dating and settle down like him. You'll see it again and again. They all mean well. They do legitimately worry about you and your well being. They are concerned about the changes they see. Yet, their thoughts and worries should be taken with a grain of salt. They're not people to look up to in the big relationship game.

Don't listen to life's losers, no matter how well-intentioned and based in love their criticisms are.

The Truly Toxic

You're very strict about what you eat. You've lost 30 lbs and you're looking really good and getting compliments from everyone. Some people you know are asking you for advice on how they can look better and be healthier, too. You become the diet, workout and weight loss guru to your little circle of friends and coworkers. Their positive feedback just gives you more energy to continue improving. The snowball effect of "positive results - feedback - more positive results" grows and grows. Things are great. And then… HE shows up. Your negative friend. *"Dude, why do you have to be such a pussy all the time? Some pizza and beer is not going to kill you."* Your friend is, of course, the quintessential "Dad Bod". He looks like a wad of bubble gum. Your improvements have given him a very real and candid look at what he COULD be with some discipline, honesty and hard work. Instead, he chooses to go with the flow and look and feel like shit. You're making it very tough for him to live in his little cocoon of a world he has built for himself. He may have even caught his wife talking about you in glowing terms and now he feels threatened. He feels that by putting you down and sabotaging your efforts, he is in-turn elevating himself. He's an asshole, in other words. Avoid him at all costs.

Let's say you're at a party with friends. It's been about a year since you divorced from your ex and you've been feeling out the dating scene for the past couple of months. Lucky for you, you've had success with the ladies of all ages and backgrounds. Your married friends live vicariously through the stories you tell of sneaking off with that gal from the coffee shop, the making out with the single MILF from the PTO meetings, the love-struck college girl who won't stop texting you, the 40-something from your office, etc. One guy from your friend group, though, doesn't take your changes too well. He's what they call the quintessential "White Knight". He takes it upon himself to stand up for the perceived damsels in distress at every opportunity. He's never met a woman he didn't put on the highest of pedestals. While most of your friends are saying that you're lucky to be getting attention from all these women, the white knight will say that you're just taking advantage of their vulnerable state and you should stop being a such a typical male predator. Nothing you or your other friends say and do will change his mind. As far as he's concerned, you represent all that is wrong with men today.

Basically, he's a little worm who can't get women and the sexual relationship he so desires. He resents those men that do have success. Him jumping on the "team woman" bandwagon is actually an underhanded and dishonest way of trying to get laid. *"If I become a super feminist, pro-female, anti-male type of man... then women will love me more"*. He's obviously wrong and he will drive himself insane with his lack of real results in life. Avoid him before his toxic ways rub off on you.

The well-intentioned can be turned around by showing them the true and positive motivations behind your changes. They're good people that are just looking out for your safety and don't want to see you get hurt. They also don't want to see you transform into something they see as truly negative. Their feelings are genuine, but that doesn't mean they aren't based on their own inadequacies. Simply maintain your mission and be there for them when they finally wake up and ask you for help in their own journey towards self-improvement (which happens more often than not).

The toxic, on the other hand, should be avoided at all costs. Nothing you say or do will transform their thinking. You shouldn't be caught up in the game of trying to win them over. The more you play into their game, the more negative you and they both become. You should instead limit as much of your time with them as possible. If possible, eliminate them completely from your life. Let them crawl back to you later. Even then, keep them at a safe distance.

Any successful man ever will tell you the same thing: **As soon as you realize your potential and start making drastic improvements to your life, the losers start coming out of the woodwork to pull you back down to their level.** Shitty people just love to try and bring others down with them. It's just an interesting quirk of human nature.

Your Habits

Your habits are all those things you do on a regular basis without even thinking about them. They are actions that, by virtue of their repetition, have just become a normal part of your day-to-day existence. They're now part of your autonomous mental programming. Many habits, as we know, are not good for you. A habit of reaching for a cigarette first thing in the morning: Not good. A habit of eating a giant fattening breakfast every morning: Not good. A habit of going out drinking after work every day with your buddies: Not good.

It took one simple decision and many days of repetition to get these habits programmed into your brain. Some habits, like cigarettes and alcohol, became habitual by virtue of their addictive chemical composition. After all, they were specifically designed and engineered to make you feel great for a short amount of time and then keep you coming back for more. There's also a social component to drinking and smoking that makes them more enjoyable and further embeds the habitual programming into your psyche. If you're happy and laughing with friends while doing it, then you're more likely to continue the behavior, lungs, and liver be damned.

Other habits aren't necessarily healthy or unhealthy, but just by doing them, again and again, they became etched into your brain. If you hang around people long enough you start to recognize their own little unique habits. Years ago, I had a coworker who had a completely unconscious ritual that he did multiple times a day. He would sit down in his office chair, grunt, grab the computer mouse, tap it twice on the desk, and then move the mouse rapidly back and forth. This was his way of waking up his computer so that he could start working. He did this every single day, multiple times a day. I didn't have to look over the cubicle wall to see if he was there, I could sit and wait for the tell-tale "grunt, tap tap, mouse-scraping" noise ritual. If you asked my coworker about his grunting tapping mouse routine, he would have no idea what in the hell you were talking about. It was all automatic. He unwittingly programmed these series of actions into his day-to-day routine. To him, it was like blinking (Now you're thinking about blinking. Sorry.).

An important key to getting over the hump in life and really achieving self-improvement is to understand and harness the power of this automated habit system we have built into all of our brains. Get control of your habits, and things happen much easier for you.

The process is two-fold:

1. Eliminate old habits that keep you from reaching your goals.

2. Do little things every day that help you achieve your goals and do

them until they become habits.

I think it's important that you sit down and take inventory of your day-to-day activities. Write it all down. Every little stupid detail, no matter how trivial, you need to write it down. If you're a complete physical disaster, your daily itinerary may look something like this:

• Wake up. Hit snooze three or four times. Get out of bed. Brush teeth. Smoke a cigarette. Drink coffee. Eat cereal. Take a shower. Put on clothes. Drive to work.

• Eat a donut or two at the office. Talk to coworkers during a cigarette break.

• Eat lunch at the pub with coworkers. Burger and fries, usually. Have a beer with meal. Smoke a cigarette afterward.

• Another cigarette break.

• Leave work. Head to the pub for a few drinks (and maybe some unhealthy food) and have at least two more cigarettes.

• Go home. Eat something. Usually something frozen or leftovers from the previous night. Maybe get fast food on the way home. Watch TV. Another cigarette.

• Take the laptop to bed. Watch Netflix or browse the internet until you fall asleep.

In the pitiful, but unfortunately realistic list above, it's pretty obvious which habits should be immediately eliminated. Smoking and drinking stick out from the list along with unhealthy eating, but so does hitting the snooze button repeatedly, going home to watch TV, and internet surfing before bed. Like for most people, there is a lot of room for improvement and it starts one habit at a time.

It's time that you identify the little day-to-day habits that need improving and do something in their place that is more positive and productive. How long until those new things you do become automated habits that you don't even need to think about? Approximately two months. Yes, you need to do something for two months before your brain finally says, "I guess we'll be filing this away in the unconscious mind and do them automatically since it's so important to you." That's when it finally clicks.

Examples of habits from the above list that can be changed:

1. Instead of hitting the snooze button, you jump out of bed immediately, quickly stretch, let out a big grunt, and run to the bathroom to take a shower.

2. Instead of eating cereal, you skip breakfast and drink coffee (thanks to your intermittent fasting routine) or eat something healthy like fruit and eggs.

3. Instead of taking cigarette breaks with coworkers, you spend the additional time doing something more productive that will help your work or take a timeout to read something you enjoy.

4. Instead of going to the pub for lunch, you bring something healthy from home and eat at your desk, or you go outside to sit in the sun and eat and chat with coworkers that also brought their lunch to work.

5. Instead of hitting the pub right after work, you go to the gym.

6. You go to the grocery store after the gym and grab something
healthy to make for dinner and for your lunches during the week.

7. You eat dinner and enjoy some downtime.

8. Instead of taking your laptop to bed, you read a book and fall
asleep at a decent time, getting as close to eight hours of sleep as
possible.

That sounds far more productive and healthier than the
alternative, but it's also not easy to do. It can all be too much to
tackle at once. I recommend you first do the obvious and eliminate
the health-killing vices like alcohol and cigarettes as step number
one. Put something else in their place immediately. Give it two
months to really sink in and make a difference.

Once those big vices are eliminated and replaced with
new healthier habits for two months, you can then start adding
on additional positive habits, but not before then. You don't want
to make the common mistake of overwhelming yourself with too
many life changes and lose something important in the shuffle.
If you throw too much on your plate at first, you will fail. People
respond better to little changes over time.

Here are some additional items you can add to your arsenal
of habits. These will all pay positive dividends down the line:

1. Go for a walk every morning.
2. Drink lots of water throughout the day.
3. Eat only fresh foods.
4. Read every day.
5. Keep a journal of thoughts and ideas.
6. Stretch every day.
7. Clean your home every day.
8. Check your personal finances every day.

9. Talk to a friend every day.
10. Do something that makes you money every day.

Every one of these habits is a step towards feeling, looking and DOING better. They all have a purpose. They're all part of a larger state of mind called "discipline". While eating pizza and staying up late watching Netflix sounds great, it doesn't do a damn thing for you. In fact, it will only help you add on weight and deprive you of the sleep you need to function properly.

There's a helpful mantra by former Navy Seal and motivational speaker Jocko Willink:

"Discipline Equals Freedom"

The only way to get to the coveted goal of true freedom in life is to have discipline in all facets of life. If you want financial freedom, then you need the discipline to take control of your finances. Don't spend frivolously. Save. Pay off debt. If you want the physical freedom that good health and energy provide, then you need the discipline to put down the snacks and beer and instead eat real foods and hit the gym. If you want the freedom of living life on your terms and the freedom to hit your goals, you say NO to the insanely hot but obviously mentally ill woman that keeps texting you. You let somebody else play the part of her savior and you focus on you, instead.

The same principles apply to life while you are in a good relationship with a genuinely good person. You use your discipline to set time for yourself and for your time together as a couple. You learn to say no to temptations and temporary pleasure that causes years of pain down the line. You recognize that a relationship is hard work and you don't give in to the notion that it "just happens".

In other words, get off your ass and do something positive. The hard work is worth it. You're worth it.

Comfort

Comfort is the enemy of all men. Keep a man well-fed, keep him entertained, and instill in him a sense of safety and security, and all of his ambition quickly goes right out the window. Marriage and having kids instill in men an instant sense of extreme comfort. We know that comfort kills a woman's sex drive, but it also kills a man's ambition. It's not a coincidence.

Woman gets comfortable and less turned on -> Man gets comfortable, lazy, and less attractive -> Women is even more turned off by the man -> Man gets no sex and is miserable -> Woman is even more turned off -> Man has even less ambition -> Woman lets herself go -> Both people are beyond miserable.

This is the comfortable death trap that so many marriages end up in.

Yes, men know they have to work, provide, and maintain the safety of the home, but it seems that today's man throws all of his eggs into the comfortable "just be a great dad" basket, and he has no time or energy left to focus on himself. Goals, ambitions, and dreams are all set aside for the greater good of the family unit. Discipline goes down the toilet, as well. The weak mindset permeates every facet of the comfortable man's life.

Being a great dad is something most good men can do in their sleep. Going beyond that and being a great MAN is something else entirely. It requires discipline and discomfort. Most men don't take the steps needed to get over the comfortable hurdles in front of them. They may have small bursts of positive energy and attempt some form of self-improvement, but the toxic people in their life do all they can to keep them in their comfortable Provider role. The men fail the mental tests thrown at them and go back into their cave of comfort.

The grand irony (there's that word again) is that we strive SO hard for comfort in our lives and that is exactly what ruins us. It takes our eye off the prize. We lose our edge. We're no longer on alert. We're no longer striving for the next best thing. We allow the warm blanket of "good enough" to hold us down. It's not until things go really bad that we realize the very real danger around us.

I often tell guys that their traumatic "holy shit" moment can be the perfect catalyst to real positive life change. Unfortunately for many, there's also a very real *"Oh God, what have I done to myself all these years?"* realization that hits and hits them hard. To realize your untapped potential is exciting... and depressing. Knowing what you could have been is sobering. Fortunately for you, there's no better time to start over than right now.

You're a man with a plan. A man with a mission. A man with a better understanding of the game of relationships. An attractive man who values himself above all others.

So... Now What?!

Epilogue

I often say you shouldn't let trauma define you as a person. This is coming from the guy who started a website, routinely writes articles about relationships, wrote two books, and started charging for consultations… all because his wife left him after a twenty-year relationship. Obviously, this was a traumatic and life-changing experience for me. But I could've taken this life in an entirely different direction. I could've started drinking way too much. I could've said to hell with it and gained 100 lbs. I could've just told my ex to take the kids full-time and ran off to California to live as a beach bum. I could've continued sleeping around with attractive but mentally ill women who would've made my life a lot more difficult. I could've killed myself.

Life gave me a pot full of really disgusting ingredients, and I've done my best to make a tasty stew out of it. I could've REALLY fucked up in a big way VERY easily. It took a lot of work to make sure I didn't. The work was well worth it. My hope is that you see YOU are worth it, too.

I've read and re-read this book countless times. I'm horrible at proof-reading (I'm sure I missed some errors here and there). I think I got across all that I intended to in an efficient manner. I could've gone on for maybe 200 more pages, but I would've lost you. You need some answers and some guidance, not countless words from a guy that likes to hear himself talk. Men like other men that get to the point.

I hope that you don't take from this book an "anti-relationship" theme. That's far from my intention. Relationships and women CAN be amazing. They can truly add to your life in immeasurable ways. After all, we human animals tend to gravitate towards pair-bonding. Even the manliest testosterone-fueled maniac has a woman on the back of his motorcycle. We all innately seem to know that going through life alone is pretty damn tough.

To have somebody by your side can make the trip a whole lot better... or a whole lot worse.

The problem is that nature also puts us in a state of mind that literally blinds us to faults that others around us see so clearly. Yes that sexy blond makes you feel like the king of the world, but she's jobless, has three kids, was once on heroin, used to have an eating disorder, and she may or may not have been a sex worker in the past. That is not a good relationship candidate. That is somebody you need to stay the hell away from.

Your Real Love partner may be out there waiting, but you may not find her. That's okay. You'll be okay on your own. In fact, you're never truly on your own. You have a brotherhood of men out there that are more than willing to extend a hand and help. The world is your oyster, my friend.

"Treat yourself like someone you are responsible for helping."

Things will work out in the end. It's all up to you. Make it happen.

Thank you for reading!!

My website:

Dadstartingover.com

Facebook group (and private group for men only):

https://www.facebook.com/dadstartingover/

Contact me:

Dadstartingover.com@gmail.com

CPSIA information can be obtained
at www.ICGtesting.com
Printed in the USA
BVHW041747180220
572699BV00012B/228